THE COMPLETE

STRETCHING

4th edition

Christopher M. Norris

B   Y

Bloomsbury Sport
An imprint of Bloomsbury Publishing Plc

50 Bedford Square   1385 Broadway
London   New York
WC1B 3DP   NY 10018
UK   USA

www.bloomsbury.com
BLOOMSBURY and the Diana logo are trademarks of Bloomsbury Publishing Plc

First published 1994; second edition 2003; third edition 2007
© Chris Norris, 1994, 2003, 2007 and 2015
Illustrations © Dave Gardner

British Library Cataloguing-in-Publication Data
A catalogue record for this book is available from the British Library.
Library of Congress Cataloguing-in-Publication data has been applied for.

ISBN: PB: 978-1-4729-0665-6
ePDF: 978-1-4729-0845-2
ePub: 978-1-4729-0840-7

2 4 6 8 10 9 7 5 3 1

Typeset in 10.75 on 13pt Adobe Caslon by Susan McIntyre

Printed and bound in China by Toppan Leefung Printing

Bloomsbury Publishing Plc makes every effort to ensure that the papers used in the manufacture
of our books are natural, recyclable products made from wood grown in well-managed forests.
Our manufacturing processes conform to the environmental regulations of the country of origin.

To find out more about our authors and books visit www.bloomsbury.com.
Here you will find extracts, author interviews, details of forthcoming events and
the option to sign up for our newsletters.

CONTENTS

ACKNOWLEDGEMENTS

My thanks go to Laura Scott-Burns, our photographer for the 4th edition of the book as well as to the models, Suzanne Roebuck and Andrea Woodhead.

I would also like to thank those involved with the previous editions, especially Jan and Peter Bowan at the Alderley Pilates Studio for providing an excellent venue for the photo shoot. Also to Susie Gale, Victoria Jones, Jean Nadin, Madge Slater, Suzanne Hattersley, who modeled for the exercises and to Grant Pritchard who took the photos.

PREFACE TO THE FOURTH EDITION

The first edition of *The Complete Guide to Stretching* was published in 1999 and since that time the book has become established as a standard text on exercise and sports courses, and an essential daily guide for users.

With each update new material has been added, layout and illustrations improved, and science base updated. For the 4th edition this process has continued, with the addition of a new chapter on Yoga. This chapter draws on the science of stretching covered in the book and applies it to these popular exercise forms.

Throughout the book, individuals are referred to as 'he'. This should, of course, be taken to mean 'he' or 'she' where appropriate.

PART **ONE**

THE SCIENTIFIC PRINCIPLES
BEHIND STRETCHING

BIOMECHANICAL FACTORS IN STRETCHING

1

The study of the effect of mechanical forces on biological materials is known as *biomechanics*. Biomechanical principles are important to all aspects of sports training, but especially to stretching. To be effective, and to prevent injury, stretching exercises must be applied on a foundation of good biomechanical principles.

LEVERAGE

The limbs and spine act as levers when we move. A lever is simply a rigid bar that moves around a fixed point called the *pivot* or *fulcrum*. Two forces act on the lever, *effort* and *resistance*. The effort attempts to move the lever, while the resistance tries to stop movement. In the body, the effort is supplied by muscle contraction, while the resistance is weight. The weight is a combination of the weight of the moving limb and the weight of any object lifted. Take as an example the arm lifting from the side of the body (*see* fig 1.1). The fulcrum is the shoulder joint, the effort is supplied by the deltoid muscle, which contracts and abducts the arm, and the resistance is the weight of the arm.

HOW DO YOU CALCULATE THE AMOUNT OF LEVERAGE?

The amount of leverage produced in any exercise can be calculated by multiplying the weight of the resistance by the horizontal distance between the point where the resistance or effort acts and the fulcrum. Figure 1.2 illustrates a simple example of a lever. A resistance of 6 kg is placed 3 m away from the fulcrum. Multiplying these together gives a leverage force of 18 units. To balance this out, the effort has to be of the same magnitude. So, the 9 kg weight has to be placed only 2 m from the fulcrum for the lever to balance.

LEVERAGE IN STRETCHING EXERCISES

It is important to note that in the example given in figure 1.2, the horizontal distance between the fulcrum and effort or resistance is used, rather than simply the distance along the lever. This means that leverage will be increased as a body-part is moved into a horizontal position, and will reduce as the body part moves away from the horizontal position (*see* fig 1.3). This fact must always be borne in mind when choosing starting positions for stretching exercises, especially with regard to injury to the spine.

Take as an example a simple toe-touching movement. Performed from long sitting, the leverage on the spine is minimal (*see* fig 1.4(a));

Figure 1.1 Leverage as the arm is abducted

Figure 1.2 Calculating leverage

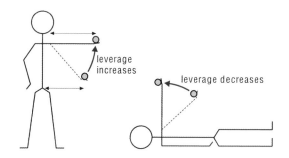

Figure 1.3 Leverage in weight training

Key point:

When calculating leverage, it is the horizontal distance from the fulcrum which is used.

however, the same body movement performed from standing (*see* fig 1.4(b)) places a considerable stress on the spine through leverage forces acting on the lumbar region.

This example illustrates an important safety factor with regard to leverage: exercises that involve moving the spine into a horizontal position will place great amounts of leverage on the spine and should be used with caution. Often, simply altering the starting position will move the spine away from the horizontal and reduce the stress on the lower back. When a horizontal position must be used, the spine should be supported. In the examples in figure 1.4, the athlete is stretching the hamstrings by bending forwards. This action places an excessive leverage stress on the spine. Simply by putting one hand down on the knee, the spine is supported and the stress reduced (*see* fig 1.4(c)).

Considering the effect of *gravity* is also important. In figure 1.5 the athlete is performing the splits. The leverage on the leg is excessive,

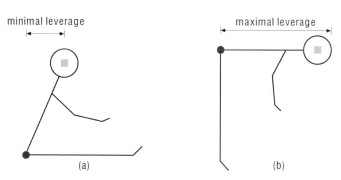

Figure 1.4 Reducing leverage by altering the starting position

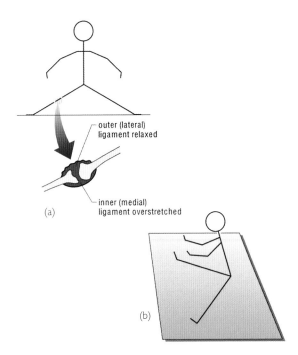

(a)

outer (lateral)
ligament relaxed

inner (medial)
ligament overstretched

(b)

Figure 1.5 Leverage and the splits (a) knees unsupported; (b) knees supported

tending to force the knee downwards, which opens the joint. This action can severely stress the medial ligament on the inside of the knee. Performing a similar action sitting down takes the weight away from the knee and, although the lever length is the same, the effect on the knee ligaments is considerably reduced, making the exercise far safer.

LEVERAGE AND POSTURE

Leverage is also important with regard to posture. A good posture (*see* page 66) is one that exerts minimal force on the joints and requires little work from the muscles to maintain it. Anything that increases either *joint loading* forces or *muscle work* can increase the risk of injury and pain, and will certainly make the posture harder to maintain over a period of time. The human body,

like any other object, has a centre of gravity, and the extension of this down to the floor is known as the *line of gravity* (*see* pages 11–12). This can be thought of as the balance point of the body's levers. When a body segment rests on this line its leverage force is minimised, and when it moves away from the line the leverage force is increased. Take as an example the head resting on the neck (fig 1.6). In a good posture, the chin is held in and the centre of the head lies directly over the neck and the gravity line. However, if the head moves forwards – as it so often does when we are looking at a computer for a long time, for example – the leverage force is increased. Using the principle of calculating leverage we can see that, if the head moves forwards, it is as though it actually weighs more. A 10 kg head resting directly over the gravity line will only weigh 10 kg, but the same head resting 20 cm forward of this line will weigh

Figure 1.6 Leverage and posture

10 x 20, or 200, units of leverage. This increased weight dramatically increases the forces on the neck and requires a significantly greater amount of muscle work to maintain it – so much so, in fact, that the muscles become tired and tight and feel knotted. The answer to this pain is simply to draw the head back on to the posture line by tucking the chin in slightly and thus reducing the leverage forces acting on the region.

CENTRE OF GRAVITY AND STABILITY

The *centre of gravity* of an object is its balance point, where all the weight of the object is focused. The centre of gravity of a symmetrical object, such as a brick, will be at its centre. However, in the case of asymmetrical objects, such as the human body, the centre of gravity will be nearer to the larger, and heavier, end.

WHERE IS THE BODY'S CENTRE OF GRAVITY?

Because the legs are heavier than the arms, when a person is standing their centre of gravity is not in the middle of the body at the navel, but lower down within the sacrum. As the body moves away from the standard upright position, the centre of gravity also moves. Lifting the arms overhead, for example, moves the centre of gravity upwards, while carrying something moves the centre of gravity towards the object being carried. In addition to the centre of gravity of the body as a whole, each limb also has a centre of gravity. For

example, the weight of the arm will act through its own centre of gravity, which, rather than being in the middle of the arm at the elbow, is actually closer to the shoulder because the upper arm is heavier than the forearm.

WHAT AFFECTS STABILITY?

Extending the centre of gravity downwards towards the floor gives us the object's *line of gravity*. Where the centre of gravity is the balance point of an object, the line of gravity can be imagined as a plumb-line hanging down from this point. For an object to remain in balance, its line of gravity must pass through its *base of support*. If the line of gravity moves outside the base of support, the object becomes unstable and will topple over.

To compensate for this, the body position will change when something is carried. In figure 1.7(a), the centre of gravity of the body is within the sacrum. In figure 1.7(b), the suitcase carried in the right hand moves the centre of gravity of the body and case combined to the right. This would move the line of gravity outside the person's base of support, making him unstable. To compensate for this, the body position is changed by leaning over to the left to pull the line of gravity back within the base of support (*see* fig 1.7(c)).

Stability is an important safety factor when performing stretching exercises. An unstable position can cause an athlete to wobble or fall, unintentionally increasing a stretch and pulling muscles or spraining joints. When discussing stability, there are two factors to consider: first,

(a) (b) (c)

Figure 1.7 The centre and line of gravity

the position of the object's centre of gravity; and second, the size of the object's supporting base.

A lower centre of gravity and a wider base of support will make an object more stable. In addition, the degree of stability is proportional to the distance from the line of gravity to the outer limits of the base of support. Take as an example a motorbike (*see* fig 1.8(a)). It has narrow wheels and thus a small base of support. In addition, the rider sits on the machine, so his centre of gravity is high. If the rider were to lean over when going round a bend, he would become less stable (*see* fig 1.8(b)). His base of support is the same, and his height above the ground is roughly the same, but his line of gravity has now moved closer to the edge of his base of support. The motorcycle rider's position is much less stable than that of a racing-car driver where the car has a wide base of support (*see* fig 1.8(c)) and, because the driver sits low in the car rather than on top of it, the centre of gravity is lower.

HOW TO INCREASE STABILITY IN AN EXERCISE?

The principles described above can be applied to the exercise situation. When performing standing exercises the centre of gravity is fairly high, so

Key point:

When performing a stretching exercise, if you are unable to balance and find that you 'wobble', first, widen your base of support in the direction of the movement and second, lower your centre of gravity.

the feet should be apart to widen the base of support, which will make the position more stable. In addition, bending the knees will lower the centre of gravity and further increase stability. When moving, the base of support should be widened in the direction of the movement, i.e. when swinging the arms forwards and backwards a wide stance should be taken with one foot in front of the other, and when moving the arms from side to side the feet should be apart. Figure 1.9 shows a variety of foot positions and their effect on stability. The narrow base (feet together, fig 1.9 (a)) is less stable than the wider base (feet apart, figs 1.9 (b-d)). In addition, where the wide base is lengthened in the direction of travel (lunge position, fig 1.9(e)), the exercise is more stable in

Figure 1.8 Stability, centre of gravity and base of support

Figure 1.9 Changing base of support and stability

Figure 1.10 Stability in stretching exercises

a forward and backward direction but less stable in a side to side direction.

In figure 1.10 the yoga position known as the tree is shown. The movement is basically a balance that stretches the adductor muscles of the hip on the bent leg. All three movements have a similar effect on the muscles, but the balance requirements are very different. In figure 1.10(a), the foot is placed on the shin and the hands are held by the sides, keeping the body's centre of gravity low. In figure 1.10(b), the foot is placed on the knee and the hands are at the chest, and in figure 1.10(c), the foot is over the hip and the hands are raised over the head. In figure 1.10(b) and figure 1.10(c), the weight of the leg and of the arms lifted above the head raises the centre of gravity of the body. The higher centre of gravity makes the position less stable and so it is harder to stay balanced.

INERTIA, FRICTION AND MOMENTUM

INERTIA

Inertia is an object's resistance to change in motion, and is proportional to its weight or 'mass'. Inertia is the force that makes a car hard to push, but a bicycle easy. The heavier an object is, the more inertia it will have. Once inertia has been overcome and the object has begun to move, less force is required to keep it in motion. This is why a heavy object may need a 'good push' to get it moving, and then, as it starts to move, it does so with a sudden jolt and seems to 'run away with itself'.

A joint possesses a certain inertia due to the stiffness (viscosity) of its synovial fluid, and the extensibility of the tissues (ligaments and muscles) that surround it. The first part of any movement sequence will often be the most difficult because it is overcoming joint inertia. Once the movement is 'going', keeping it going is often easier. The first action in any set of stretches can be seen as a warm-up, and each subsequent movement will gradually increase in range. In addition, a warm joint will offer less resistance to movement in general, and its inertia will be less. A warm-up before stretching, or before any sport that involves a range of motion exercise, is therefore important.

FRICTION

Friction, on the other hand, is the force that tries to stop one object from sliding over another. Frictional forces are the result of roughness on the surfaces of two opposing objects and can be reduced with the use of a lubricant, like oil or water. On a rubberised floor, the roughness of the floor and the sole of the shoe produces a large amount of friction and gives considerable grip. A shiny wooden floor produces less friction, and a patch of water will reduce friction still further and may cause a person to slip and fall.

MOMENTUM

Momentum is the combination of how heavy an object is and how quickly it is moving (mass and velocity). A heavy object, such as a leg or the trunk, which is moving quickly will possess a lot of momentum and will be very difficult to stop. The high degree of momentum can take over the movement so that the athlete is no longer able to control it: this is when injuries can occur. To reduce the likelihood of injury through momentum, rapid actions should only be performed in mid-range. When going to full range, actions should be slow and controlled to avoid damage to the joint structures and to muscles. Momentum is a particularly important factor in both dynamic and ballistic stretching (*see* pages 59–60).

> **Key point:**
>
> When prescribing stretching exercises with movement (dynamic or ballistic actions) consider the effects of momentum on the body tissues.

TENSION, COMPRESSION AND SHEAR

Tension, *compression* and *shear* are all examples of mechanical stresses that can act on the body, causing the body tissues to deform.

Tension is a pulling force. When the spine is flexed, the spinal ligaments are tightened and subjected to a tension stress that causes them to lengthen.

Compression stress is the opposite to tension stress. It is a pushing force, applied along the length of a tissue. When a person is standing upright, the knee cartilages (menisci) take the weight of the body and compression stress is applied to them, causing them to flatten.

Shear stress occurs when opposite forces are applied to a tissue, causing one part of the tissue to slide over the other. For example, if an athlete who is running stops suddenly by digging their foot into the ground, shearing stress is applied to the knee. Bodyweight tries to keep the athlete moving forwards, but – because the foot is fixed on the ground – the ground force pushes in the opposite direction. The result of these two opposing forces is shear.

MECHANICAL STRESSES AND INJURIES

Both compression and tension stresses act in line with the tissue fibres, in the direction in which the tissues are strongest. Shearing stresses, however, are imposed at an angle to the fibres, making this type of stress potentially the most dangerous in terms of injury. For example, a fall on to a straight leg will exert a compression stress on the joint structures. These forces will be largely absorbed, unless they are very severe. During the fall, tension stress will be imposed on the muscles if the joints bend, and the elastic capabilities of the muscles will take some of the stress away from the joint. Falling at an angle will again cause some compression and tension, but shearing will also take place between the body tissues and the foot and ground. This type of stress can cause injury, and a fracture may result.

TISSUE REACTION TO LOAD

THE LOAD–DEFORMATION CURVE

When a load is applied to a body tissue, the tissue will deform. The relationship between load (stress) and deformation (strain) can be represented graphically by the load–deformation curve (*see* fig 1.11). Initially, when the load is applied the tissue demonstrates elasticity. The

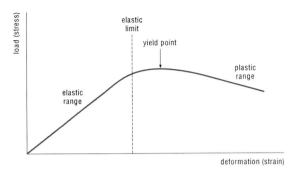

Figure 1.11 The load–deformation curve

deformation of the tissue at this point of the curve is directly proportional to the load that is applied (a relationship known as Hooke's law). As the load is released, the tissue returns to its original shape – it literally 'bounces back'. To begin with, the amount of deformation is proportional to the load applied and there is said to be a *linear relationship* between load and deformation along this part of the curve called the *elastic range*.

If the load continues, the tissue is stretched beyond its elastic range and a point is reached at which deformation becomes permanent. Past this point, known as the *elastic limit*, the tissue will not return to its original shape when the load is released, and a permanent change will occur. Instead of acting in an elastic fashion, the material is now said to be *viscous* or *plastic* in its reaction to load. The more load that is applied, the more deformed the material becomes. Instead of returning the load and bouncing back, the tissue is absorbing and dampening some of the load.

Eventually, the yield point is reached, at the highest point of the curve. After this point the material continues to deform even though the load applied to it is not increasing; this means severe damage is occurring to the body tissue. This behaviour – continued deformation with constant load – is known as *creep*.

PROPERTIES OF BODY TISSUES

Body tissues combine both viscous and elastic properties, so they are *viscoelastic*. One of the essential features of the deformation of viscoelastic materials is that it is time dependent. This means that when a load is applied rapidly (sudden stretch) the deformation will be elastic, and the tissue will spring back. If the load is applied for some time (stretch and hold) the deformation becomes viscous, and the tissue will slowly 'give'.

COMPOSITION AND RESOLUTION OF FORCES

COMPOSITION OF FORCES

In figure 1.12(a), two men are pulling on ropes attached to a car bumper. A man pulls at 45 degrees to the car (force A); another also pulls at 45 degrees but on the other side of the car (force B). The net result is that the car rolls forwards. This process demonstrates the *composition of forces*. The forces supplied by the men pull at 90 degrees to each other, combining to produce a third force – the *resultant* – which pulls the car forwards. If both of the original forces (called *component* forces) are equal, the car will move forwards in a straight line. However, if the right-hand force is greater than that on the left, the car will still move forwards, but it will veer off to the right.

A similar effect occurs in the body when two muscles pull to create a third force. For example, when the quadriceps muscles are pulling on the patella, the vastus medialis pulls inwards, and the vastus lateralis pulls outwards. The result is a centrally directed pull of the kneecap. However, if one muscle is substantially stronger or tighter than the others, the direction of the patella will change and pain may result.

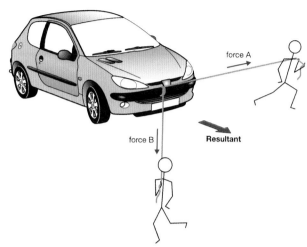

Figure 1.12(a) Forces A and B combine to produce the resultant

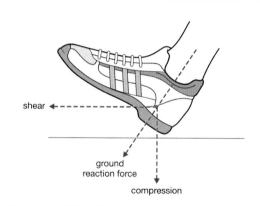

Figure 1.12(b) The ground reaction force has two components: shear and compression

Key point:

When performing a stretch, do not just consider the actual movement that is occurring, but the forces that combine to produce it as well.

RESOLUTION OF FORCES

Where we have just one force, we can use the reverse process to obtain the two original forces which make up the resultant. Now we are using the process of *resolution of forces* to more accurately demonstrate the effect of the force on the body. For example, when someone who is running places their foot on the ground a force known as the *ground reaction force* is created. This acts obliquely to the ground (*see* fig 1.12(b)). This single force may be resolved into its two components: one of which acts vertically to create compression or jarring stress on the foot; and one of which acts horizontally, causing shearing or friction on the foot.

COMPOSITION OF FORCES IN STRETCHING EXERCISES

The composition of forces can also be important when performing stretching exercises. Take as an example the quadriceps (or rectus femoris) stretch (*see* page 107). As we bend the knee, the top of the patella is pulled upwards along the length of the femur and the patella tendon pulls downwards, in the opposite direction. The result is a composition of these two forces to create a third force compressing the patella on to the femur below. This action can be very painful for someone suffering from inflammation of the front of the knee (*see* fig 1.13).

DESCRIBING BODY MOVEMENT

AXES AND PLANES

For descriptive purposes the human body may be divided into three planes. The *sagittal* plane passes through the body from front to back, dividing it into right and left halves. The *frontal* plane divides the body into anterior and posterior sections,

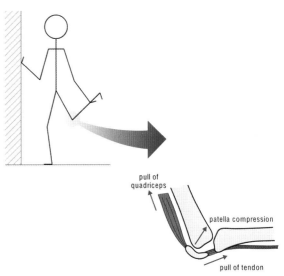

Figure 1.13 Patella compression can be very painful

and lies at right angles to the sagittal plane. The *transverse* plane divides the body into upper and lower portions, and rests at right angles to the other two planes.

Each of the three body planes has an associated axis which passes perpendicularly through it (*see* fig 1.14). Movement occurs in a plane but about an axis. Abduction and adduction occur in the frontal plane about an antero posterior (AP) axis; flexion and extension occur in a sagittal plane about a transverse axis; and rotations occur in a transverse plane about a vertical axis.

In reality, movements do not just occur in one plane, but in several. This is because a complex series of movements link together to give a motion that occurs in all three planes about an oblique axis.

ANATOMICAL TERMINOLOGY

Standard terminology should be used when describing body movements to avoid confusion. For example, instead of 'bending' we use flexion, and instead of 'straightening' we use extension.

vertical axis

sagittal
axis

frontal
axis

transverse
plane
(rotation)

sagittal plane
(flexion/
extension)

frontal plane
(abduction/
adduction)

Figure 1.14 Axes and planes

To describe the position of part of the body, we again use standard terminology. So, instead of saying 'in front' we use the term anterior, and instead of 'above', the term superior is used.

Figure 1.15 shows the common terms used to describe movement and the position of the body.

RANGE OF MOTION

The *range of motion* (ROM) of a muscle refers to the length of the muscle at any point in a movement. *Outer range* is from a fully stretched position to the mid-point of the movement. *Inner range* is from this mid-point to a fully shortened position of the muscle. *Mid-range* is an area

between these two extremes and is the region in which most everyday actions occur (*see* fig 1.16).

It is important that the body tissues are regularly taken through their full range of motion to maintain their extensibility and elasticity. When this does not occur, the muscle can shorten permanently, completely altering the function of a joint. For example, in a sedentary individual it is common for the hip flexors to become shortened, because most everyday movements only work these muscles within their inner range. The shortened muscle may then pull on to the lumbar spine, giving back pain.

SUMMARY

- A lever is a rigid bar that moves around a fixed point called the fulcrum.
- Leverage is calculated by multiplying the horizontal distance between the fulcrum and the line of action of a force acting on the lever.
- Keeping body parts close to the posture line reduces the effects of leverage.
- The centre of gravity of the body is near the sternum.
- When exercising, stability can be increased by lowering the body's centre of gravity (bending the knees) and widening the base of support (standing with the feet apart).
- As a body tissue is loaded, initially its reaction is elastic (it springs back) then plastic (it permanently deforms).
- Forces may be resolved into two components acting at 90 degrees to each other.
- Motion may be outer, mid-, or inner range.

Figure 1.15 Anatomical terminology

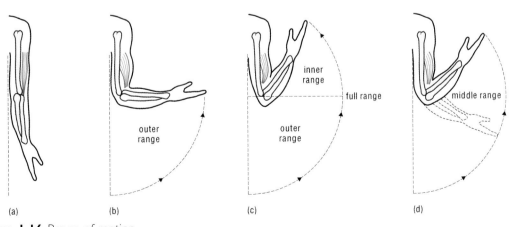

Figure 1.16 Range of motion

JOINT STRUCTURE AND FUNCTION

BONES

The body has over 200 separate bones. Each is a rigid structure made from calcium, phosphorous and proteins. Bones may be divided into four major categories: long, short, flat and irregular.

- **Long bones** are the type found in the limbs such as the thigh (femur) and upper arm (humerus). Their primary use is to act as levers for the muscles to pull on when producing movement.
- **Short bones** are cube-shaped and seen in the carpels of the hand and tarsals of the forefoot.
- **Flat bones**, such as the scapulae and ribs, form broad areas for muscle attachment and serve to protect vital organs of the body.
- **Irregular bones**, such as the vertebrae, protect and support the body.

HOW DO BONES FORM?

Bone begins life as cartilage in the foetus. During the second month of pregnancy the cartilage bone begins to change into bone proper by a process known as *ossification* (*see* fig 2.1). This begins in an area in the middle of the bone known as the *primary* centre and gradually spreads towards the bone-ends. This central portion of ossified bone is called the *diaphysis*, while the end of the bone which is still made of cartilage is the *epiphysis*. During adolescence, a *secondary* ossification centre appears in the epiphysis. Ossification here spreads towards the shaft, leaving a thin cartilage growth plate (epiphyseal plate) sandwiched between the two regions of ossified bone.

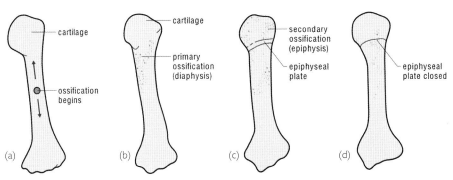

Figure 2.1 Ossification of centres in the bone: (a) embryonic (b) infancy (c) adolescence (d) mature

HOW DO BONES GROW?

The growth plate is responsible for change in the length of the bone. As a person reaches maturity, the epiphyseal plate will disappear and the shaft and extremity of the bone fuse into one solid unit. The epiphyseal plate is an area of potential weakness in the young bone, and, if damaged, can result in permanent deformity of the bone. This is especially true of the upper part of the femur in sport, and great care must be taken when giving stretching exercises to children so that excessive strain is not imposed on the hip.

> **Key point:**
>
> When giving stretching exercises to children to work their muscles, consider the effects that these same movements are having on their growing bones.

WHAT ARE BONES MADE OF?

As a long bone ossifies, its shaft becomes a cylinder with hard compact bone on the outside surrounding a central medullary cavity. The bone cavity contains bone marrow, responsible for making blood cells. The epiphysis is made from spongy cancellous bone with a thin compact bone covering. The other bone types do not contain a cavity, but instead are made up of a honeycomb of cancellous bone with a thin compact bone covering. This makes them light, although they may be bulky.

JOINT TYPES

In order for movement to occur in the body, the bones must articulate. The point at which this occurs is called a joint, and consists of two bones separated by various types of tissue. The shape of the bone-ends involved in a joint will dictate how much movement can occur, and which movement types are allowed. Joints may be broadly classified into three major groups, known as *fibrous* (immobile), *cartilaginous* (slightly mobile) and *synovial* (freely movable) (*see* table 2.1).

FIBROUS JOINTS

Fibrous joints allow little, if any, movement. Examples include the joints formed between the bones of the skull (a *suture* joint), those of the teeth (*gomphosis*), and *syndesmosis*, an example of which is found between the upper end of the fibula and the upper outer aspect of the tibia.

The edges of the bones forming the suture joints of the skull are jagged and separated by fibrous tissue. This type of joint will not normally allow any perceptible movement, and may close up completely after the age of 30. The syndesmosis is also separated by fibrous tissue, but contains more than the suture joint. The fibrous tissue in this joint forms a ligament that allows small amounts of twisting and stretching movements. The gomphosis consists of a peg which fits tightly into a socket and is held in place by a fibrous band.

CARTILAGINOUS JOINTS

In cartilaginous joints, the bones are separated by a pad of cartilage tissue, and both primary and secondary types exist. The primary cartilaginous joint has articular cartilage separating the bones. They occur as the growth plates at the ends of bones in children. At the beginning of adult life, the growth plate closes and the two pieces of bone (the diaphysis and epiphysis) become one bone. The secondary cartilaginous joints are found in the centre line of the body; examples include the spinal discs and the joint between the two pubic bones (known as the *symphysis pubis*). The bone-ends of the joint are separated from each other by a fibrocartilage pad, a structure which allows limited movement.

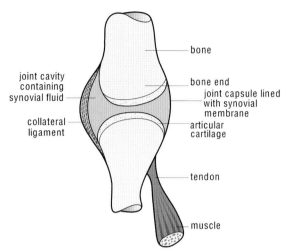

Figure 2.2 Typical synovial joint structure

Figure 2.3 Accessory movements in a joint

SYNOVIAL JOINTS

The synovial joints are the ones we are most concerned with when using stretching exercises. They move freely and contain a variety of joint structures. A typical synovial joint consists of two bone-ends covered by articular cartilage (*see* fig 2.2). The joint is surrounded by a fibrous joint capsule. Certain portions of the capsule are thickened to form supporting ligaments. The capsule is lined with a thin synovial membrane that secretes a lubricating liquid called *synovial fluid*. Structures inside the joint or within the capsule are known as *intracapsular*. Structures associated with the joint but found outside the capsule are called *extracapsular*. These include small balloon-like pads or bursae, which stop structures rubbing over each other, and small 'fat pads' that fill the gaps between tissues.

Muscles control the joint, and those passing close to the bones may attach some fibres to the joint structures. For example, the popliteus muscle of the knee also attaches to the medial knee ligament and medial knee meniscus.

There are seven main types of synovial joints (*see* fig 2.3).

The plane joint has relatively flat surfaces and permits gliding or twisting of one bone against the other. The intertarsal joints of the foot are examples of plane joints.

The saddle joint has one convex surface and one concave surface arranged at right angles to each other, as with a horse rider sitting in a saddle. The major movements occur in two planes, with a slight amount of combined movement occurring in a third plane. An example is the carpometacarpal (CMC) joint of the thumb.

The hinge joint allows movement in one axis only, and a strong joint is formed with tight ligaments. An example is the elbow joint (humeroulnar), formed between the humerus and ulna.

The pivot joint allows a rotation movement about one axis only. One piece of bone rotates in a ring formed by the other bone and ligament tissue. An example is the joint formed between the radius and the ulna in the elbow (superior radioulnar).

The ball and socket joint allows movement in all three planes, examples being the hip and shoulder joints. A ball-shaped surface of one bone articulates with a cup-shaped surface of the other.

The condyloid joint is similar to the ball and socket, but allows movement in only two planes. The metacarpophalangeal (MCP) joints of the fingers are examples.

The ellipsoid joint is again a modification of the ball and socket. The convex surface of one bone is oval in shape, while the concave surface of the opposing bone is elliptical. The radiocarpal joint in the wrist is an example here.

JOINT STRUCTURES

INDIVIDUAL DIFFERENCES IN JOINT STRUCTURES

Although each person has the same joint types, there is tremendous variation in the general structure and function of joints between any two individuals.

The shapes of the bones will vary. This can be due to hereditary influences, physical training or injury. Some people are naturally more, or less, flexible because of the shapes of their bones.

Those who have exercised regularly since an early age will be considerably different from inactive individuals. For example, girls who have spent many years practising ballet as children will tend to be more flexible around the hips for the rest of their lives.

Injury and disease will also affect the range of motion possible at a joint. Older athletes who have varying amounts of arthritis will show reduced movement in specific patterns. For example, lateral rotation of the shoulder and hip tends to be very limited. Where an injury has occurred early in life, the growth plate in a bone may have been affected. A severe fall from a bicycle or horse can often dislodge a bony growth plate and alter the formation of the final mature bone.

The structural differences at a joint must be appreciated when comparing ranges of movement between individuals. Even with the same amount of training, two people may never gain the same amount of movement at a joint.

CONNECTIVE TISSUE AND THE FORMATION OF JOINT STRUCTURES

The tissues of the body are of four basic types (*see* table 2.1). *Epithelial* tissue consists of densely packed cells that form coverings, and make up skin and the outer coating of organs. Connective tissue (described below) consists of loosely arranged cells. *Muscular* tissue has the ability to contract, and nervous tissue to conduct electrical impulses.

Connective tissue is composed of cells floating within a fluid known as an *extracellular matrix*. The composition of the cells and matrix determines the type and function of the particular connective tissue described. The cells have many functions including creating and maintaining the fluid matrix and ultimately breaking it down. Three types of fibres are found within the matrix. *Collagen* fibres are the most abundant and are so profuse that they may form one third of the total bodyweight. The collagen fibres have a rope-like appearance and are strong but non-elastic. The second type of fibre found is *elastin*. This resembles a coiled spring and has great elastic capacities. The elastin fibres

Table 2.1	Tissue types
Tissue	**Function**
Epithelial	Tightly packed cells which form coverings and make up skin and the outer coating of organs
Connective	Loose cells in fluid base which modify to form joint structures
Muscular	Contracts muscles
Nervous	Conducts electrical impulses

crisscross each other to form a net, similar to the springs in a bed mattress. The third type of fibre is *reticular* fibre. Reticular fibres are really a type of collagen, and are very fine fibres that branch to form a meshwork.

The basic design of connective tissue is modified to form the various joint structures described below.

TYPES OF JOINT STRUCTURES
Articular cartilage

The ends of the bones forming a joint are covered by articular (hyaline) cartilage, a modified connective tissue. The cartilage matrix contains specialised cells known as *chondrocytes*, which maintain its integrity. It also contains both collagen and elastin fibres in varying proportions together with proteoglycan, a protein that acts as a sponge to trap water, giving cartilage an exceptionally high (70–80 per cent) water content. Cartilage has no blood vessels or nerves, relying instead for its nutrition on the synovial fluid. Substances move into and out of the cartilage by diffusion from the synovial fluid, a process heavily reliant on regular movement to cause alterations in pressure within the fluid. As the cartilage is compressed intermittently with movement, for example walking or running, nutrients are pumped into and out of the cartilage. With continuous loading, such as occurs in prolonged standing, the cartilage is compressed further and further without allowing more fluid to be taken up. This continual compression without release can reduce the cartilage depth by as much as 40 per cent.

The area of cartilage next to the bone (the sub-chondral region) is firmly attached to the bone and will resist shearing stresses. The main body of the cartilage contains fibres that will resist tension stresses, while the fluid within the cartilage gel resists compression stresses. The fibres are elastic, and the gel will gradually

Key point:

Articular cartilage relies on regular movement for its nutrition. Without movement it will degenerate.

flow away from any compressing force. It is the combination of these two reactions that gives cartilage a viscoelastic property.

The joint capsule

The joint capsule is composed of two parts. The outer portion (*stratum fibrosum*) is tough and fibrous, and is thickened in certain areas to form ligaments. The inner portion of the capsule (*stratum synoviale*) is loose and contains many blood vessels. This region blends with the synovial membrane of the joint.

The capsule is attached to the bones around the edge of the joint, and at the line of attachments many small blood vessels are seen. The capsule has a rich supply of nerve fibres responsible for the 'joint sense' (proprioception) used in balance and reflex actions. The capsule is particularly important after injury. Following joint sprains, the joint will swell, and the accumulation of fluid will stretch the capsule causing tightness and pain. After injury, the capsule can thicken and further limit the joint movement, requiring specialist physiotherapy techniques and regular stretching exercises to regain the lost movement.

When capsular tightening limits movement at a joint, not all movement directions are reduced equally. The joint becomes swollen, increasing the volume of fluid contained within the capsule and its lining synovial membrane. The increased fluid volume and pressure leads the joint to take up a position of ease; that is a position which reduces intra-capsular pressure. The capsular

Key point:

Following injury to a joint, the capsule may be tight, requiring clinically oriented stretching exercise.

Table 2.2	Capsular patterns of common joints
Joint	**Pattern of limitation (1 most, 2 less, 3 least)**
Shoulder	1. Lateral rotation 2. Abduction 3. Adduction
Elbow	1. Flexion 2. Extension
Wrist	1. Equal of flexion and extension
Hip	1. Medial rotation 2. Flexion and abduction 3. Extension
Knee	1. Flexion 2. Extension
Ankle	1. Plantar flexion 2. Dorsiflexion
Lumbar spine	1. Extension 2. Equal limitation to side flexion 3. Flexion*

* where limitation to the lumbar spine is due to facet joint (synovial joint) rather than disc (fibrous joint).

pattern is dictated by muscle action, and the shape and extent of the capsule. Its presence demonstrates to a therapist that there is an acute swelling within the joint. Each capsular pattern is specific to a joint and the limitation is of a fixed proportion (measured as a ratio) rather than total amount (measured in degrees). For example in the knee joint there is a greater limitation of bending (flexion) than straightening (extension), and for the shoulder joint outward turning (lateral rotation) is the most limited movement. Table 2.2 lists the capsule patterns of common joints.

Synovial membrane

The synovial membrane lines the joint capsule and consists of two distinct layers. The inner layer secretes the synovial fluid, while the outer layer is a loose, highly vascular structure consisting of collagen fibres and fat cells. This outer layer merges with the membrane covering the bones, the *periosteum*.

The blood vessels of the joint divide into three branches: one travelling to the epiphysis at the end of the bone; the second to the joint capsule; and the third to the synovial membrane itself. The blood vessels contained in the synovial membrane can exchange fluid and nutrient molecules with the synovial fluid. The synovial membrane has a series of folds in it and, as the joint moves, it will unfold like a fan to allow movement (rather than simply stretching). The folds of the synovial membrane have extensive lubrication to virtually eliminate friction.

Ligaments

Many ligaments are simply parts of the joint capsule that have thickened to resist particular stresses on the joints. They are made of connective tissue fibres, and attach to the bones of the joint. The ligament fibres are arranged along the lines of stress imposed on the joint. As a joint moves, the ligaments will stretch, initially pulling the fibres straight and then stretching them. Exercise will regularly lengthen the ligaments and strengthen them, but stretching exercises that overstress the ligaments should be avoided. The ligaments support the joint, and, if overstretched, can leave the joint too flexible, causing it to be insecure and open to injury. Following a ligament injury, it is particularly important to keep the joint moving gently, so that the newly healing ligament fibres will again align themselves correctly, rather than in a haphazard fashion.

Ligaments at the side of the joint (collateral ligaments) resist stresses which would tend to open the joint sideways. Other ligaments are positioned to protect the joint in its most vulnerable movements. For example, in the knee the cruciate ligaments prevent the thighbone (femur) from sliding forwards and backwards on the shinbone (tibia), and in the shoulder the glenohumeral ligament prevents the ball of the shoulder (head of humerus) from moving too far forwards in its socket (glenoid) and dislocating.

Consideration must be given to ligaments when stretching at all times. Stretches that are excessive or brutal in their application may actually damage the ligamentous support of a joint and cause severe injury.

Key point:

Many ligaments are simply thickened parts of the joint capsule.

Muscle–tendon unit

The muscles are attached to the bones via a tendon. This is an inelastic collagen structure that simply transmits the force created by the muscle to the bone in order to move it. The tendon is able to transmit the force to a small area, keeping the bulk of the muscle away from the joint. Some tendons, such as those of the finger muscles, are very long, allowing the muscles to be positioned in the forearm, well away from the finger joint where the muscle force is applied. Other tendons, such as that of the deltoid muscle of the shoulder, are right next to the muscle itself.

The thick, central part of the muscle is called the muscle belly, and it is this part that bulges as the muscle contracts. The muscle then tapers down towards the tendon and this area between the muscle and tendon is called the musculo-tendinous junction. The tendon then inserts into the bone via the teno-osseous junction.

Definition:

The musculo-tendinous (MT) junction is the join between the muscle and tendon, the teno-osseous (TO) junction is between the tendon and bone.

FASCIA

Muscle is contained within a framework of connective tissue called *fascia*. The fascia forms compartments (*see* page 202) that contain the contractile fibres of the muscle itself. If you were to take a piece of muscle and dry it by removing all the water, the dry powder that would remain represents the building blocks of the muscle. Although most of us think of muscles as giving strength and contracting to lift weights for example, in actual fact the dry weight of the contractile proteins of a muscle is about equal to the dry weight of the non-contractile material. In other words, there is as much non-contractile fascia within a muscle as there is contractile tissue!

So what does all this fascia do? In addition to providing the framework that holds the muscle together, fascia can actually create force, not through contraction but through elastic recoil. As you stretch a muscle, it will spring back or recoil partly because of the elasticity of fascia. In addition, some muscles attach to bones not via tendons, but by tendinous sheets of fascia each called an *aponeurosis*. In this case, the fascia transmits some of the force created by the muscle. Finally, between each major muscle, the fascia is thickened into a structure called the *intermuscular septum*. This is the thick white 'marbling' that you see in meat when you cut it across.

Although muscles are each separate structures, their fascias are joined together into a tough fibrous network. In some areas, these fascias become specialised and have a specific name attributed to them. In the back, for example, there is the thoroco-lumbar fascia (TLF), and on the outside of the thigh there is the iliotibial band (ITB). The importance of fascia from the point of view of stretching is that a stretch will often affect several muscles at once, all of which are linked by fascial pathways or 'tracts'. To describe the effect of movements on both the muscle and fascia at the same time, we use the term *myofascia*, meaning the contractile muscle fibres and the fascial framework surrounding it.

Key point:

When designing stretching exercises for individual muscles, consider that the various muscles may actually be linked together in myofascial tracts.

LUBRICATION OF JOINT CARTILAGE

The articular cartilage has no blood supply. As we have seen, it relies largely for its nutrition on materials being passed from the synovial fluid. Movement will flush fresh fluid over the cartilage surface, and alterations in pressure will press nutrients into the cartilage. If the joint does not move properly, for example following injury, nutrient material may not be pressed into the cartilage, and that area may subsequently degenerate, giving osteoarthritis.

The synovial fluid provides a lubricating mechanism that cuts down the amount of friction the joint is subjected to. As the two bony surfaces move over each other, the small synovial fluid molecules act as tiny ball-bearings preventing the opposing cartilage surfaces from rubbing away. Some of the fluid is absorbed into the cartilage almost like water in a sponge. As pressure is exerted on the joint, for example when standing or walking, the fluid is squeezed out of the cartilage to form a fluid film that separates the cartilage surfaces and again prevents them rubbing.

It is often said (usually by inactive individuals) that exercise causes arthritis. This is far from the case. Movement will actually keep the joint cartilage healthy and is essential for the general health of the joint. However, if an injury occurs and an athlete tries to 'train through the pain', the biomechanics of the joint will be altered and changes may occur in the joint cartilage, ultimately leading to the development of arthritis. In addition, a balance must be kept between the strength of muscles supporting a joint and the flexibility of the joint structures. If a person becomes too flexible, the joint will not be secure. Similarly, if a person has too little flexibility, their joints will be stiff. Either case will alter the normal biomechanics of a joint and could give problems later in life.

Key point:

Joint cartilage needs regular movement to give it nutrition and keep it healthy.

JOINT MECHANICS

PHYSIOLOGICAL AND ACCESSORY MOVEMENTS

Two major types of movement are possible at any joint. First, there are the normal actions that an athlete controls, such as flexion and extension. These are known as *physiological* movements. But there are also *accessory* movements, which cannot be produced directly but occur automatically as a joint moves, giving 'joint play'. For example, as the knee bends and straightens, the femur and tibia will also glide and roll on each other. The bending and straightening (flexion and extension) are the physiological movements, while the gliding and rolling are the accessory movements. Three distinct types of accessory movements occur, known as roll, slide and spin.

Roll is similar to a car tyre rolling over the road surface. At any point, the same areas on the tyre will be in contact with the same areas on the road surface (*see* fig 2.4(a)). If slide occurs, a single point on one surface will be in contact with a number of other points on the opposing surface, as when a car tyre skids (*see* fig 2.4(b)). Spin occurs when both points on the two opposing surfaces are in contact, and pure rotation occurs as with a 'spinning top' (*see* fig 2.4(c)).

Accessory movements become important to general flexibility after injury. If a joint is stiff, stretching it will regain the physiological movements but may not bring back the accessory movements. This can leave the joint feeling awkward and open to injury. For this reason, it is always wise to see a physiotherapist after suffering a sports injury to have the joint movement properly assessed.

CLOSE AND LOOSE PACK

The two opposing surfaces of a joint do not fit together exactly – they are said to be *noncongruent*. However, with the joint in one particular position its surfaces will come as close together as they are able, and this is known as 'close pack'. In this position the joint capsule and ligaments twist and pull the joint surfaces tightly together. The joint space is at a minimum, the concave surface of one bone fits closely on to the convex shape of the other, and no further movement is possible. In the close-pack position, stress will be taken on the bones in a fall because the ligaments in a joint are fully tightened and unable to 'give' any more. A fracture is often the result.

The loose-pack position is exactly the opposite. As the joint surfaces are released from their close-pack position, elastic recoil of the soft tissues surrounding the joint enables its surfaces to move apart, maximising the joint space. The joint will be less secure in this position and more movement will be possible. Should the athlete fall with the joint in a loose-pack position, the joint will often move too much, and ligament injury can result.

Figure 2.4 Accessory movements in a joint

Key point:

A loose-pack position, where the joint structures are relaxed and the joint surfaces have moved apart slightly, will facilitate free movement.

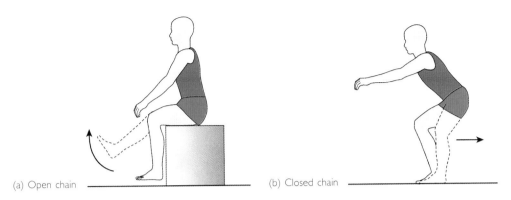

(a) Open chain   (b) Closed chain

Figure 2.5 Open and closed chain actions

OPEN AND CLOSED CHAIN MOVEMENTS

OPEN CHAIN ACTIONS

An open chain action occurs when the end joint in a limb (terminal joint) can move freely, as when the foot is off the ground or the hand is off the wall. In a closed chain movement the end joint is unable to move freely because the foot is on the floor or the hand is on the floor or wall, and part of the bodyweight is taken through it (*see* fig 2.5). Open chain actions are often rapid movements such as punching and kicking where the limb can move freely and rapidly (called a *ballistic* action). Here, muscles begin the movement and end it, but the middle part of the action also relies on the momentum of the moving limb. You are literally throwing the limb into the action.

CLOSED CHAIN ACTIONS

Closed chain actions are generally slower movements requiring co-contraction of muscles; that is muscles on either side of the joint (agonist and antagonist) working together. In closed chain actions the joint is loaded (compressed) and the muscle work occurs to stabilise the joint.

When planning a programme it is important to identify which actions are open chain and which are closed chain, because the demands on joints, muscles and tissues will be different for each.

SUMMARY

- There are over 200 bones in the body, each made from calcium, phosphorous and proteins.
- Most bones begin life as cartilage and harden through a process of ossification.
- Synovial joints are surrounded by a capsule strengthened by ligaments.
- When a joint is injured, movement is limited in a capsular pattern.
- The joint contains synovial fluid, and the bone ends are covered by cartilage.
- Joints need regular movement to stay healthy.
- Joints have two types of movement: physiological and accessory.
- Physiological movements consist of bending, straightening and twisting, while accessory movements give the joint its healthy spring.
- In the close-pack position a joint is tightly locked, whereas in the loose-pack position it moves freely.
- In an open chain action the joint is unloaded by bodyweight, in a closed chain action the joint is loaded.

29

// MUSCLE ACTION

3

HOW MUSCLES WORK

Muscle contraction itself is more important to strength training than to stretching. However, because stretching is primarily affecting muscle, it is vital that we have some understanding of the general principles underlying muscle actions.

STRUCTURE OF A MUSCLE
Muscle membranes

If we take a small piece of muscle tissue and magnify it many times (*see* fig 3.1(a)), we can see that it is made up of many long muscle fibres. Each individual muscle fibre is surrounded by a thin membrane (*endomysium*), and in turn the fibres are grouped together in bundles covered by the *perimysium*. Finally, the whole muscle structure is encased in a sheath, the *epimysium*.

The muscle membranes stretch the whole length of the muscle from tendon to tendon, intimately linking the contractile and inert portions of the muscle. The whole structure is often referred to as the 'musculo-tendinous unit'. The muscle membranes are part of the fascia (*see* pages 201–203). This not only encases the muscles, but actually spreads across and between muscle groups linking them together in fascial pathways.

The combination of fibre contraction and elastic recoil of the muscle membranes is important for the development of 'elastic strength' (*see* page 32). Therefore, stretches that target myofascial pathways are important for speed and power sports involving the whole body, such as martial arts and dance.

> **Key point:**
>
> Muscle membranes link several muscles together and are important in the development of 'elastic strength'. They should be considered when stretching for power sports in particular.

Muscle microstructure

A further membrane, the *sarcolemma*, surrounds the individual muscle cells. The sarcolemma is important because it is electrically conductive; it has within it *sarcoplasm*, a fluid containing fuel stores (*glycogen*) and enzymes important to muscle contraction. Within the sarcoplasm is an intricate membrane, the *sarcoplasmic reticulum*. This membrane contains transverse tubules, each of which end on the muscle cell surface as a lateral sac.

Looking closely at each fibre, we see alternating light and dark bands, corresponding to different muscle proteins. The light area is composed of a thin filament called *actin*, while the dark area consists of a thicker filament called *myosin*. The

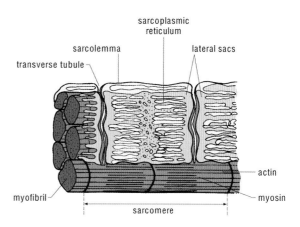

Figure 3.2 Structure of a muscle – transverse tubule system

Figure 3.1 Structure of a muscle – contractile mechanism: (a) whole muscle and group of muscle fibres; (b) myofibril; (c) sarcomere; (d) thick and thin filaments

HOW DO MUSCLES CONTRACT?

Contraction of the muscle occurs when the muscle filaments move towards each other, and a whole sequence of events is required for this to take place. When we want a muscle to contract, a nervous impulse is sent from the brain. This impulse travels down the spinal cord and along a peripheral nerve to the muscle, where it causes changes on the surface of the muscle fibre. At the point where the nerve touches the muscle, a chemical (*acetylcholine*) is released, which causes an electrical impulse to spread across the surface of the sarcolemma. As a result, calcium is released from the lateral sacs and passes down the transverse tubule to bind with the troponin molecule (*see* fig 3.2). This reaction causes the spiral tropomyosin to move deeper into the groove of the actin filament removing the inhibition. Once the inhibition has been removed, contraction will occur spontaneously, and the muscle filaments pull closer together, causing them to slide over each other and shorten the muscle.

The whole muscle contraction process uses energy, and rest is needed to recharge the structures involved. Calcium has to be moved out of the transverse tubule of the muscle and

two sets of filaments fit together like the fingers on two opposing hands, one set of actin–myosin fibres being called a *sarcomere*. The thick myosin filament has projections or 'crossbridges' coming from it, much like the oars of a boat. The thin actin filament has a long *tropomyosin* filament wound around it and a globular *troponin* molecule is positioned over this area. At rest the tropomyosin prevents (inhibits) actin and myosin from binding.

back into the lateral sacs. The filaments must then return to their original relaxed positions.

WHAT AFFECTS MUSCLE STRENGTH?

The amount of overlap that can occur between the sliding filaments of the muscle will determine its *contractile strength*, and the relationship between muscle length and tension development is called the length–tension relationship (*see* fig 3.3). When the muscle is shortened, the filaments are overlapped already and have little additional movement available to them. In the shortened position (inner range), therefore, the muscle is comparatively 'weak'. In the lengthened position (outer range), the filaments have pulled apart and the actin and myosin elements are disengaged. Again the muscle is relatively 'weak' – it can produce little active force through contraction – however, because the muscle is now stretched, it is able to produce some force through elastic recoil, known as elastic strength. Therefore, the force in the outer range is mostly created passively through recoil, rather than actively through contraction.

It is only in mid-range, when the muscle filaments are engaged but not overlapping, that maximal active force can be developed. Mid-range is the range that we mostly use in our normal day-to-day activities, so functionally it is appropriate that this should be the strongest point in the available movement.

Definition:

Contractile strength results from muscle contraction, while elastic strength comes from muscle recoil as a result of elasticity in the stretched muscle and reflex mechanisms.

MUSCLE REFLEXES

Three muscle reflexes are important when using flexibility training: the *stretch reflex*; *autogenic inhibition* (also known as the reverse stretch reflex); and *reciprocal innervation*.

STRETCH REFLEX

The *stretch reflex* is important both for postural control and muscle tone. It relies on information coming from special receptors called *muscle spindles* (*see* fig 3.4(a)). The muscle spindle is a cigar-shaped structure attached alongside the main muscle fibres. When the muscle is stretched, so is the muscle spindle. The stretch of the spindle is detected by nerves, and a reflex occurs that causes the muscle to contract and shorten the spindle once more.

The stretch reflex reacts to change in both the length of the muscle and in the velocity of its movement. Change in length is important for postural or *tonic* control, while change in velocity is important for movement or *phasic* control. The classic example of the stretch reflex acting for phasic control is the knee jerk, or patellar reflex. Here, the patella tendon is stretched rapidly by being hit with a small rubber hammer. This rapid stretch is picked up by the muscle spindles in the

A = overlap of muscle filaments
B = maximum tension when filaments aligned
C = muscle overstretched (filaments pulled apart)

Figure 3.3 Length–tension relationship of a muscle

Figure 3.4(a) Muscle receptors

quadriceps and causes nerve impulses to be sent to the spinal cord. Impulses return from the cord to the quadriceps causing them to contract, and the knee straightens quickly giving a small 'kick'.

The stretch reflex is also essential for the maintenance of normal standing posture through tonic control. When we stand up we continually sway forwards and backwards. As we start to fall forwards, there is a pull on our calf muscles, changing their length and causing a stretch reflex. The calf muscles then contract a split second later to pull us back to the upright position again.

The reflex occurs in three parts (*see* fig 3.4(b)). The first response is a short latency contraction (M1), which results from activation of the spinal reflex circuit itself. The second response is a long latency contraction (M2), which involves the

lower centres of the brain. The third response, (M3), occurs occasionally and is again a result of brain activity rather than the spinal cord. Voluntary contractions can occur within 170 milliseconds of the detection of a movement, but the stretch reflex occurs much faster. M1 occurs within 30 milliseconds and M2 within 50–60 milliseconds. The stretch reflex therefore causes muscle contraction in response to an unexpected stretch some 140 milliseconds (nearly one-fifth of a second) before voluntary muscle contraction.

The result is that the stretch initiates a contraction of the same muscle that limits the stretch itself, creating a negative feedback system sometimes referred to as a *resistance reflex*. The reflex is protective, tending to stabilise a joint, and relies on a continuous barrage of nerve impulses coming from the joint itself. This process is known as 'joint sense' or *proprioception*.

After injury, these nerve impulses can be lessened (proprioception is impaired) tending to make a joint less stable. Therefore, an essential part of sports rehabilitation is the use of training to increase the number of nerve impulses being fed to a joint. This is achieved by performing a large variety of movements, especially those which tax balance skills, as these will feed more and

Figure 3.4(b) Muscle activity during the stretch reflex occurs in three phases

more nerve impulses into the joint. This type of training, known as proprioceptive exercise, will help to restore the stability of a joint by improving the 'reaction time' of the muscles supporting it. In this way the stretch reflex is restored to its correct level of action and it is able, once more, to support the joint.

> **Key point:**
>
> Proprioception is often impaired following injury, and needs to be retrained using special exercises based on balance and stability.

AUTOGENIC INHIBITION

Another receptor, the *golgi tendon organ* (GTO), is situated in the muscle tendon (*see* fig 3.4(a)). This receptor measures tension. When a muscle contracts, it shortens, so a stretch reflex will not occur. However, the GTO will register the increasing tension in the muscle tendon and will then cause a reflex relaxation of the muscle, a process known as *autogenic inhibition*. This is the reverse situation to the stretch reflex and has a protective function, preventing the muscle from contracting so hard that it pulls its attachment off the bone. The two reflexes do not occur at the same time, because the threshold of the GTO is set far higher than that of the muscle spindle. In normal everyday movement, tension in the muscle is not high enough to cause autogenic inhibition.

Both stretch and autogenic inhibition reflexes have important implications for stretching exercises. Stretching that involves short jerking movements will tighten the muscle through the stretch reflex, while sustained stretching (over about 30 seconds) will allow the muscle to relax. Relaxation occurs because the stretch reflex becomes desensitised, and, if the muscle tension is high enough, autogenic inhibition follows through stimulation of the GTO. The autogenic inhibition in this case overrides the stretch reflex.

RECIPROCAL INNERVATION

A further reflex is called *reciprocal innervation*. This occurs when the antagonist muscle relaxes to allow the prime mover to create a movement. For example, when the biceps muscle contracts to bend the elbow, the triceps will relax through reciprocal innervation to allow the movement to occur. This reflex can be used to obtain further relaxation in a muscle just prior to stretching.

> **Key point:**
>
> The stretch reflex increases muscle tone in response to muscle stretch, autogenic inhibition reduces tone when tension detected in a tendon is too great and reciprocal innervation relaxes a muscle when its neighbour contracts.

ELASTIC AND CONTRACTILE PROPERTIES OF MUSCLE

Muscle has three properties: contractibility, elasticity and extensibility.

CONTRACTIBILITY

The contractile nature of muscle results from the movement of the sliding filaments within the muscle fibre.

Isometric

When the actin and myosin filaments come together, force is generated and the muscle will shorten. If the muscle filaments shorten, but the external length of the muscle remains the same, the muscle tenses but the joint on which the muscle works will not move. This is an *isometric* or static muscle contraction. An example is holding an object in the hand with the elbow bent to 90°.

Concentric

When the muscle filaments shorten and pull the attachments of the muscle closer to each other, causing movement at the joint, the muscle contraction is then *concentric*. In our example above, instead of the arm being held still, the elbow joint flexes. A concentric action tends to accelerate a limb. The movement begins slowly and gets faster.

Eccentric

Once the elbow has been flexed, and the muscle filaments shortened, lowering the weight again involves the muscle filaments slowly paying out to control the joint as it extends. This is an *eccentric* action. This type of action is used to slow the body down and control movements such as sitting down into a chair or coming downstairs. Each time, the muscle filaments are sliding apart and the muscle is lengthening.

> **Key point:**
>
> In isometric contraction the joint does not move; concentric contraction causes acceleration; and eccentric contraction causes deceleration.

ELASTICITY

Individual muscle fibres are grouped together in bundles (*see* page 30) and each fibre is surrounded by a connective tissue sheath (the endomysium).

Figure 3.4(c) Flexion–relaxation response: (a) body is lowered by eccentric activity of the back muscles; (b) at full flexion the back muscles are fully stretched; (c) recoil of the stretched muscles begins the upward trunk movement – no muscle contraction is required initially

The bundles themselves are again aligned in groups and surrounded by another sheath (the epimysium). The muscle sheaths cannot contract, but they will stretch, and they have important elastic properties. These elements of the muscle are known as the *parallel elastic components* because they are aligned parallel to the muscle fibres. The tendons at the end of the muscle are also non-contractile, but again they show elastic properties. These are the *series elastic components*, so called because they are positioned before and after the fibres.

We know that there is a linear relationship between load and elasticity from the load–deformation curve (*see* page 15). As we load a muscle it will stretch proportionally, and, as the stretch ceases and the muscle springs back, energy is released.

EXTENSIBILITY

If the stretch is applied slowly and released slowly, so that the muscle remains relaxed (non-contractile), the force produced by the muscle is purely passive. This is especially important in posture. As we bend forwards to touch our toes, the back muscles (erector spinae) are lengthening eccentrically to lower the trunk. However, these same muscles are also being placed on stretch. When we begin to come back up from the forward bend position, initially there is no muscle contraction. We begin our upward movement purely through elastic recoil of the back muscles, a process known as the flexion–relaxation response (*see* fig 3.4(c)). This mechanism is simply a way of conserving muscle

energy, but it does illustrate the importance of maintaining healthy elasticity within a muscle. For example, if a person suffers from chronic low back pain, the flexion–relaxation response no longer occurs because the back muscles are continuously in spasm and are unable to relax and stretch. The result is that the muscles have a poor blood flow (because blood no longer pumps through the muscle as it contracts and relaxes) and acids build up in the muscles, causing pain.

As stretches become more rapid, the force produced is a combination of both elastic and contractile properties. When we lengthen a muscle its filaments move apart, ready to contract once more, and the elastic elements of the muscle are stretched. If this stretch is applied rapidly, a stretch reflex occurs, causing the muscle to tighten and pull against the stretching force. If the muscle contracts immediately afterwards, the contractile force produced will be a summation of contraction, elastic recoil, and reflex mechanisms and will be far greater than if the muscle contracted from rest (*see* fig 3.5). This type of pre-stretching is used

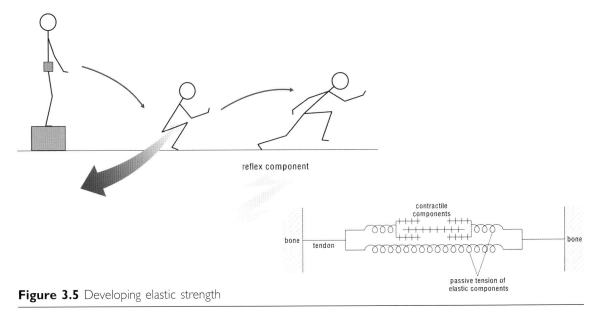

reflex component

bone

tendon

contractile components

bone

passive tension of elastic components

Figure 3.5 Developing elastic strength

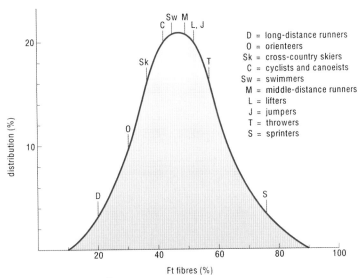

Figure 3.6 Distribution of fast twitch fibre types

MUSCLE FIBRES

TYPES OF MUSCLE FIBRES

All muscles contain fibres of different types. Red fibres are designed to contract over and over again without fatiguing, and are known as *slow-twitch* fibres. White fibres are called *fast twitch*, and these give short bursts of power. A person's muscles will contain both fibre types, but in different proportions. Those who are good at endurance sports tend to have more slow-twitch fibres in the leg muscles, while those who perform explosive sprints have more fast-twitch fibres (*see* fig 3.6).

ARRANGEMENT OF MUSCLE FIBRES

No matter which type is present, each muscle fibre is only able to shorten and reduce its length by half. Although the same amount of shortening occurs with each fibre, altering the arrangement of these fibres within a muscle will affect muscle function. Two different arrangements are found, one for short powerful muscles and the other for long flexible ones.

The short powerful type is like the deltoid muscle of the shoulder. Here, the fibres are arranged side-by-side, inserting into a central tendon like the barbs on a feather. There are many of them so the muscle is very powerful. However, the fibres are short so the muscle cannot move very far and is therefore comparatively inflexible. This type of arrangement is called *pennate* (*see* fig 3.7(a)).

Long slender muscles like the hamstrings on the back of the leg have their fibres arranged parallel to each other, attaching to tendons at each end (*see* fig 3.7(b)). This type of muscle is called *fusiform*. There are fewer fibres, so the muscle is less powerful. However, the muscle will still shorten by half, and, as this type of muscle is much longer, the movement it produces will be of a greater range. When choosing

Figure 3.7 Arrangement of muscle fibres: (a) shorter fibres of pennate muscle; (b) longer fibres of parallel fusiform muscles

stretching exercises it is important to be aware of the underlying muscle structure to devise more effective programmes.

If we are throwing an object or hitting a ball we often need to develop the maximal amount of force possible. The amount of force will be dependent on our underlying strength, but also on the flexibility of a muscle and on the range of motion through which a limb is taken. This is because when we are able to use a greater range of motion, we have more time to allow the speed of an object to build up. Take as an example the javelin throw. If an athlete has very stiff shoulders, he or she will not be able to take the javelin very far back. An athlete with good flexibility around the shoulders will be able to develop greater force by accelerating the javelin for a longer period.

Key point:

Pennate muscles, being short and stocky, are built for power. Fusiform muscles are long and slender, producing high levels of mobility.

GROUP ACTION OF MUSCLES

A muscle can only pull, it cannot decide which action to perform. We produce an infinite variety of actions with a finite number of muscles by combining the various actions in different ways. This coordinated action of the various muscles working on a body-part is called the *group action of muscles* (*see* table 3.1).

PRIME MOVER (AGONIST)

When a muscle pulls to create a movement it is said to be acting as a *prime mover* or *agonist*. Most muscles can take on this function, depending on the action required and the site of the muscle. Other muscles may be able to help with the action, but are less effective than the prime mover. The muscles that help are called **secondary** or **assistant movers**. If we take elbow flexion as an example, both biceps and brachialis can flex the elbow. In most circumstances, the biceps is more effective and so acts as the prime mover, with the brachialis as the secondary mover.

ANTAGONIST

The muscle that would oppose the prime mover if it is contracted is known as the antagonist. If we bend the arm, the biceps will act as the prime mover to create the power necessary to carry out the movement. To allow the movement to occur, however, the opposite muscle – in this case the triceps – must relax and in so doing acts as an antagonist (*see* fig 3.8).

STABILISER (FIXATOR)

Muscles do not simply create movements; they are also able to stabilise parts of the body or prevent unwanted actions by acting as *stabilisers* or *fixators*. In this case, the muscle will contract to steady or support the bone on to which the prime mover attaches. Take as an example the sit-up exercise. The abdominal muscles attach

Table 3.1	Group action of muscles (example: elbow flexion)			
Prime mover (agonist)	**Secondary (assistant) mover**	**Antagonist**	**Stabiliseor (fixator)**	**Neutraliser**
Creates primary movement (*biceps*)	Assists prime mover (*brachialis*)	If contracted, would oppose prime mover (*triceps*)	Stabilises or fixes bone origin of prime mover (*shoulder muscles*)	Removes unwanted action of prime mover (*pronators*)

from the ribcage to the pelvis, so when they contract they will move both body areas, tending to posteriorly tilt the pelvis and pull the ribcage down. To allow the abdominals to contract more effectively, we need to fix one body area to provide a firm base for the muscles to pull on. This occurs by the hip flexor muscles acting as fixators to stop the pelvis from tilting as the abdominals contract. In the case of elbow flexion, mentioned above, because the biceps attach to the shoulder girdle, these bones must be stabilised to stop them sliding on the ribcage as the biceps contracts.

NEUTRALISER

Many muscles can perform more than one movement. In the case of the biceps, for example, as well as flexing the elbow the muscle can also twist the forearm upwards (*supination*). If we want the biceps to perform just one action, bending the arm but not twisting it, other muscles must contract to stop the biceps from twisting the forearm. These muscles, which eliminate unwanted actions, are acting as *neutralisers*. As we saw above, the biceps muscle cannot decide which action to perform and which not to perform. Again it must be emphasised that a muscle can only pull: if we want to alter the action it will produce, we must bring other muscles into play as neutralisers.

(a) biceps contracts as the prime mover (agonist) to flex the elbow

triceps acts as antagonist and relaxes

(b) abdominal muscles pull on ribcage and move pelvis simultaneously

hip flexors fix pelvis, enabling abdominals to pull on a stable base

(c) muscle A flexes and rotates bone clockwise

muscle B neutralises this rotation action by rotating bone anticlockwise

Figure 3.8 Group action of muscles: (a) prime mover/antagonist; (b) fixator; (c) neutraliser

TWO-JOINT MUSCLES

Some muscles cross over two joints, and are said to be *biarticular*. The hamstrings, for example, attach from the seat bone (ischial tuberosity) to the top of the tibia. Because they cross both the hip and knee joints they are capable of creating, or limiting, movement at both joints. Other biarticular muscles include the rectus femoris and gastrocnemius in the lower limbs, and the biceps and triceps in the upper limbs. Biarticular muscles have a number of important biomechanical features.

PASSIVE INSUFFICIENCY

First, because they pass over two joints, they cannot shorten enough to allow full movement at both joints simultaneously. For example, with the knee bent and the hamstrings relaxed at the knee, the hip can flex maximally enabling the knee to be pulled right up on to the chest (*see* fig 3.9). However, with the knee straight, and the lower portion of the hamstrings stretched, hip flexion is more limited. This limitation of movement at both joints is called *passive insufficiency*.

ACTIVE INSUFFICIENCY

If you stand up and flex your hip, you will be able to bend your knee actively to touch your buttock with your heel. If you pull your hip into extension first, however, and try the same movement, you will find that you are unable to touch your heel to your buttock. This is because in the first example the upper portion of the hamstrings was lengthened and the lower part shortened. In the second example, the upper and lower parts of the muscle are unable to shorten fully at the same time. This inability to create full movement at both joints simultaneously is called *active insufficiency*.

> **Key point:**
>
> A two-joint (biarticular) muscle such as the hamstring or rectus femoris does not permit full movement at both of the joints it spans at the same time.

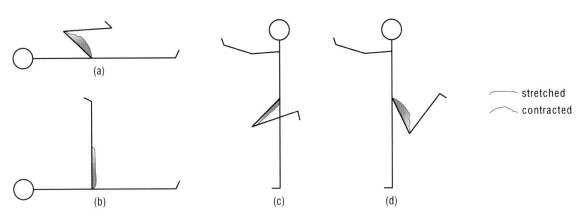

stretched

contracted

Figure 3.9 Active and passive insufficiency of a muscle: (a) hamstring stretched at the hip but relaxed at the knee; (b) hamstrings stretched over both joints (passive insufficiency); (c) hamstring stretched at the hip and controlled at both joints (active insufficiency); (d) hamstrings contracted at both joints (active insufficiency)

CONCURRENT MOVEMENT

Because biarticular muscles are unable to permit full movement at both joints at the same time, the tension in one muscle will cause tension to build up in its antagonist. For example, if the hamstrings contract and extend the hip, they will stretch the rectus femoris which is acting as an antagonist. The stretch in the rectus will then tend to pull the knee straight and extend it. When both the hip and knee are extending in this fashion, *concurrent movement* is said to be occurring. If we look at what happens to the muscle, we can see that this type of action actually conserves energy. The hip and knee are both extending, so the hamstrings are shortened at their upper end and lengthened at their lower end. The rectus femoris is shortened at its lower end and lengthened higher up. This action has therefore avoided both active and passive insufficiency, by neither shortening nor stretching both ends of either muscle. It is used in running as we push off from the ground.

COUNTERCURRENT MOVEMENT

In a kicking action the opposite occurs. When the hip is flexed and the knee extended, both the upper and lower portions of the rectus femoris are shortened, while both parts of the hamstrings are lengthened. The rectus therefore rapidly loses tension while the hamstrings rapidly gain tension, an example of *countercurrent movement*.

Key point:

When the two points covered by a biarticular muscle move in the same direction (i.e. extension–extension), concurrent movement is taking place. When they move in opposite directions (i.e. extension–flexion), the movement is countercurrent.

MUSCLE IMBALANCE AND CORE STABILITY

Muscles can be broadly categorised into two types, depending on how they function in day-to-day activities (*see* table 3.2). Some muscles, for example gluteals, act as postural or *stabilising* muscles, while others, for example hamstrings, act as locomotion or *movement* muscles.

Table 3.2	Muscle imbalance
Stabilising muscles (postural)	Movement muscles (locomotion)
Characteristics	Characteristics
Deep	Superficial
Predominantly slow-twitch	Predominantly fast-twitch
Single joint	Two-joint
Reduced activity (inhibited)	Preferential recruitment
Lengthen	Tighten
Light resistance	High resistance and ballistic
Correction	Correction
Improve tone and endurance	Stretch the tight muscles

STABILISING MUSCLES

Stabilising muscles tend to be placed deeply within the body and act as postural muscles. Examples include the deep abdominals (transversusabdominis) and the deep spinal muscles (multifidus), as well as the gluteals in many situations (*see* table 3.3). These muscles are built for endurance and have many slow-twitch fibres. They contract minimally, but hold the contraction for a long time. Unfortunately, in a person with an inactive lifestyle, or in someone who is active but has poor alignment,

Table 3.3	Examples of muscle types	
Stabilising muscles	**Movement muscles**
Deep abdominals	Superficial abdominals
Gluteals	Hamstrings
Vastus medialis	Rectus femoris
Soleus	Gastrocnemius
Serratus anterior	Pectoralis major
Lower trapezius	Latissimus dorsi

the stabilising muscles often have very poor tone and tend to sag. They almost seem to 'give way to gravity'. The tone is poor in these muscles not because they are weak, but because the nerve impulses, which control all muscles, find it difficult to get through to the muscle, and we say that the muscle has poor recruitment.

The poor recruitment of the muscle occurs because the muscles have been infrequently used, and often because a person has had pain. For example, when a person has knee pain, one of the stabilising muscles of the knee (vastusmedialis) will waste, and the same is true of other regions of the body. When we have back pain, our deep abdominals and our deep spinal muscles tend to waste and the nerve impulses to these muscles are reduced. Because the muscles have not been used, we find it difficult to switch them back on – it is a case of 'use it or lose it'.

Key point:

Stabilising muscles react to injury by demonstrating poor recruitment. Their level of tone is low and they take on a sagging appearance.

MOVEMENT MUSCLES

Movement muscles, on the other hand, tend to be more superficial, for example the hamstrings on the back of the thigh and rectus femoris on the front. These muscles are very active in sport, being our sprinting and kicking muscles. They work over two joints, in this case the knee and hip, and tend to get very tight and powerful as they are recruited by hard and fast exercise and heavy poundages such as in weight training.

Muscles of this type appear firm to the touch (palpation) and are often painful and hard after long periods of static posture, for example in sitting or standing. They commonly develop focal pain areas known as *trigger points* (TrP) (*see also* page 96). When touched firmly, the TrP can cause the muscle to contract rapidly and 'jump' or 'flick' painfully. In addition, pressing the TrP can cause pain to travel (refer) along the length of a limb. For example, a TrP in the buttock when pressed firmly cause pain to spread across the buttock and down into the thigh. TrPs around the scapula commonly give pain across the shoulder and down into the arm. The pain can be intense and burning in nature. There are several methods of releasing a TrP, one of the most effective being stretching, either passively or using the PNF techniques described on pages 61–62.

CORRECTING THE IMBALANCE

Because many forms of training tend to involve harder and faster movements, i.e. 'going for the burn', rather than slow controlled actions, for example yoga and tai chi, we end up with an imbalance of muscle length and tension around a joint. The imbalance leaves us with tight, strong superficial muscles on the one hand and sagging, poorly toned, deeper postural muscles. This gives rise to a number of postural problems and leaves us open to muscle injury through tearing. To correct the imbalance we must do three things:

Key point:

Movement muscles tend to be tight and may be painful, developing sore focal areas called trigger points.

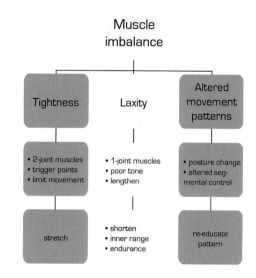

Figure 3.10 The muscle imbalance process

stretch the tight muscles; improve the tone and endurance of the postural muscles by shortening them; and correct any alignment problems which have occurred (*see* fig 3.10).

To begin with we must work for core stability. This involves tightening the abdominal muscles to provide a stable base before we begin stretching. If we fail to do this, as we stretch our alignment may be very poor. In figure 3.11, the subject is trying to stretch the rectus femoris muscle on the front of the thigh by flexing the knee and extending the hip at the same time. To do this, the pelvis must remain stable, and must not move. However, in this diagram the subject has been unable to hold the abdominal muscles tight enough to stop the pelvis from tilting forwards. They are unable to stabilise the lumbo-pelvic region. The stress from this exercise is therefore thrown on to the lower back, potentially causing back injury. For this reason, learning to stabilise the lumbo-pelvic region is essential before lower limb stretching exercises begin. This technique is described on pages 74–75.

Enhancing stability is the start of a longer process of muscle imbalance correction. However, in order to correct the sagging stabilising muscles, we must ultimately shorten them, as excessive length rather than poor strength is their major problem. This is achieved by working the muscle only in its inner range rather than in its mid- or outer range. Inner-range work is paralleled with endurance exercise using exercises known as *inner range holding* – literally taking the muscle into its

inner range and building up holding time. Instead of adding weight progressively (2 lb, 4 lb, 6 lb etc.), as would be done in weight training, we progress holding time (2 seconds, 10 seconds, 30 seconds etc.).

Stretching forms the major part of the management of the shortened movement muscles in the imbalance correction process, and a variety of techniques is covered in the later sections of this book.

Finally, when a person's body has been in a state of imbalance for a long period, the body learns inappropriate *movement patterns* and these must be corrected. Such patterns include bending the back rather than the knees when lifting, hitching the hip when moving the leg sideways and shrugging the shoulder when lifting the arm into abduction. The underlying problem is one of coordination of one part (segment) of the body when moving another, and correction of this process is known as *segmental control*. Modification of general muscle imbalance is out

Figure 3.11 Stretching the rectus femoris (a) Normal pelvic tilt and lower back alignment; (b) pelvis moves excessively, causing lower back to hollow; leg goes higher, but technique is faulty

of the realm of this book, and we shall be focusing on stretching the tight movement muscles only. The interested reader is referred to Norris, C. M., (2001), *Abdominal Training: enhancing core stability* (2nd edition), A & C Black, for a user's manual and Norris, C. M., (2000), *Back Stability*, Human Kinetics, for a textbook for therapists.

SUMMARY

- A muscle is made up of actin and myosin filaments, which slide together causing the muscle to contract.
- There are three muscle reflexes relevant to stretching: the stretch reflex, autogenic inhibition and reciprocal innervation.
- Muscle demonstrates contractability (pull), extensibility (stretch) and elasticity (spring).
- Muscles consist of slow-twitch fibres built for endurance and fast-twitch fibres, which are built for power.
- A muscle that creates a movement is a prime mover (agonist); the muscle that relaxes to allow a movement to occur is the antagonist.
- A muscle may also hold a body part firm (stabiliser) or prevent an unwanted secondary action (neutraliser).
- A biarticular muscle works over two joints.
- Stabilising muscles tend to become lax and sag; movement muscles tighten.
- Muscle imbalance may result in inappropriate movement patterns.

PRINCIPLES OF TRAINING

4

WARM-UP

Before starting any exercise session, it is essential to warm up. There are two main reasons for this: first, warming-up can make sports injuries less likely in certain circumstances; second, the body works more efficiently when warm and sports performance may actually improve. A good warm-up will have physiological, mechanical and psychological effects.

PHYSIOLOGICAL EFFECTS

It takes some time for the body to change from its basic 'tick over' at rest to a point at which it is ready to perform maximally. If vigorous exercise is started immediately from rest, the heartbeat is speeded up with a jolt instead of increasing gradually, and the beats of the heart can become irregular, rather than showing their normal smooth rhythm. These changes affecting the heart can be potentially very serious in the older or less active individual, and especially in those with a history of heart or circulatory problems.

Effects on the heart

In 1973 an important study was conducted which showed the importance of a warm-up to the cardiovascular system (Barnard et al., 1973). Researchers took a group of men with no history of heart problems and made them run vigorously on a treadmill for 10–15 seconds without a warm-up. In 70 per cent of these subjects, abnormal changes were seen on an electro cardiogram (ECG) machine. These changes, called ischaemia, showed that insufficient blood was getting to the heart muscle, a potentially very dangerous situation. However, when the same subjects ran on the treadmill after performing a warm-up, the ECG changes were greatly reduced, and in many cases the trace was completely normal, demonstrating considerably less strain being imposed on the heart. In addition, blood pressure (BP) was taken when the subjects ran on the treadmill both with and without a warm-up. Average blood pressures of 168 mmHg were taken in those subjects who ran without a warm-up, while for those who did a warm-up the blood pressure averaged 140 mmHg, some 12 per cent lower. Again, these changes demonstrate the importance of a warm-up in reducing the strain placed on the heart by vigorous exercise.

Key point:

A warm-up will reduce the strain placed on the heart by vigorous exercise.

Effect on body tissue

A warm-up will allow the body tissues to work more efficiently. Normally, while relaxed, the muscles receive only about 15 per cent of the total blood flow. The rest goes to the body organs such as the brain, liver and intestines. During vigorous exercise, because the muscles need far more fuel to provide energy, their requirement for blood increases and they need 80 per cent of the total blood flow. It takes time to re-route this blood by opening some blood vessels and closing others, and if the muscles are required to perform maximally before the blood flow has changed, they will work inefficiently.

Incidentally, this process of alteration in regional blood flow is the reason why you should not exercise within an hour of eating a heavy meal. After eating, we need the blood to stay in the region of the stomach and intestines to effectively absorb the digested foodstuffs. If we start to exercise during this period, much of the blood will move away from the digestive organs and into the working muscles. The result can be digestive upsets and 'stomach cramps'.

Key point:

Changes in regional blood flow mean shunting blood from the body organs to the exercising muscles. A warm-up makes this process smoother and more graduated.

Lactic acid formation

The body can produce energy by two methods: aerobically (with oxygen) and anaerobically (without oxygen). The aerobic method is preferable, because when we work anaerobically we produce a waste product called lactic acid. Unfortunately, we cannot work aerobically straightaway as it takes time to switch the aerobic system on. If we start intense exercise without a warm-up, the aerobic system does not have enough time to switch on; we therefore have to provide energy anaerobically, with resultant lactic acid formation.

The function of a warm-up is to 'switch on' the aerobic system and allow the body to reach a steady state where the energy provided by the body exactly matches its requirements through exercise. Once this is done, less waste is produced and so our recovery after exercise will be much faster.

MECHANICAL EFFECTS

The mechanical effects of a warm-up occur as a direct result of tissue heating. Chemical reactions involved in the production of energy for the working muscle and the removal of waste products are speeded up with warmth. In addition, nerve impulses travel faster when a nerve is warm. The effects of a warm-up on nerve conduction is particularly important for the speed of reflexes, which protect the muscles from injury.

When a substance is heated it becomes more pliable, and this is exactly the same for the body tissues. We have seen that there is a relationship between load and deformation of a tissue (*see* fig 1.11). One of the effects of a warm-up is to move the load–deformation curve to the right. This means that, for any given load, a warm tissue will be elastic for longer and will reach its failure point later. The effect of these changes is to make stretching exercises both more effective and safer. In addition, the fluid within a joint becomes less stiff (viscous) when warm so the joint will move more smoothly.

Figure 4.1 shows the effect of heat on a tendon as it is stretched. Because tissues will stretch more easily after a warm-up, it is important that stretching exercises are not performed at the beginning of a warm-up period. Vigorously touching the toes will not act as a warm-up for the hamstrings, and may tear them instead!

(a)

(b)

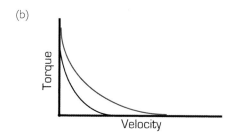

Figure 4.1 Vertical jump test – effect of tissue temperature increase due to a warm-up: (a) peak power increases, demonstrated by the increased height; (b) maximum velocity of shortening increases, and torque–velocity curve shifts to the right (from Enoka, 1994)

Key point:

A warm-up enables the body to reach a 'steady state' of energy production gradually, and makes tissues more pliable and ready to exercise.

PSYCHOLOGICAL EFFECTS

Two effects are important here: *arousal level* and *mental rehearsal*.

Arousal level

There is a direct relationship between arousal and performance, and this can be illustrated on the *human performance curve* (*see* fig 4.2). Initially, as arousal increases, so does performance. However, after a certain point an individual becomes too aroused (they are now 'stressed') and their performance suffers. As an illustration of this mechanism, imagine you have had a boring day and you arrive at the gym not really wanting to exercise. Your arousal level is low so your exercise performance will be poor. If you then go into an exercise class, however, the instructor, the music and the other people will increase your arousal level. You feel motivated and your exercise performance improves. On the other hand, imagine you are an athlete competing in an important game and you miss a shot that normally you would find very easy. Perhaps you are nervous, your heart is pounding and your arousal level is too high, so your performance suffers.

The function of a warm-up should be to place an individual at the optimum point on the human performance curve; this will change depending on the individual and the sport. A person who is very introverted and under-aroused may need to be 'psyched up' in a warm-up to move them to the right on the curve. Someone who is aggressive, extrovert and 'hyperactive' may need to be calmed down and moved further to the left on the curve. Events that require highly skilled movements tend to be performed better at lower levels of arousal

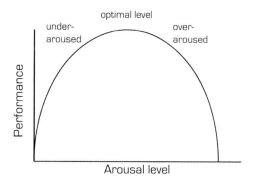

Figure 4.2 Human performance curve

when an individual is calm and can focus his or her attention. Events that require power or explosive actions are normally performed better when higher levels of arousal are achieved. This is why stretching exercises are best performed after a gentle but thorough warm-up to heat the body tissues, but relax the mind.

> **Key point:**
>
> A good warm-up will make a person optimally aroused for sport. An anxious individual should be calmed down and an under-motivated one should be 'psyched up'.

Mental rehearsal

The second psychological effect of a warm-up is that of mental rehearsal. Complex actions tend to be forgotten between exercise bouts. The first or second repetition of a complex action may not be as good as the fourth or fifth, when we have had time to 'get into' the movement. With skilled actions, it is essential that we rehearse the movement, slowly going through a golf swing, for example, before we perform the action at full speed. This is very important with activities that require a high degree of active flexibility, such as dance and martial arts.

TYPES OF WARM-UP

A warm-up can either be *passive*, with the body heated from the outside, or *active*, using exercise to form the heat internally. An example of a passive warm-up is to have a sauna or hot shower. An active warm-up can be achieved through gentle jogging or using light aerobics. Both types of warm-up can be effective, but are appropriate in different situations.

An active warm-up is the type normally used before exercise, while the passive warm-up is useful when stretching a muscle tightened from a previous strain. The advantage of the passive warm-up, from the point of view of injury, is that it does not require the athlete to move the injured tissues in order to create body heat. The use of external heat can also reduce pain and muscle spasm, helping the muscle to relax and allowing the stretch to be taken further.

In addition to active and passive types, a warm-up may also be either *general* or *specific*. A general warm-up, such as jogging or static cycling, will affect the whole body. The effects here are mainly on the major body systems such as the heart, lungs and blood vessels. This should be followed by a specific warm-up concentrating on the body part and action to be used in a particular exercise. The effects now are more localised, mainly affecting body tissues used in the actual exercise and rehearsing the action to be performed (*see* fig 4.3).

WARM-UP TECHNIQUES

The amount of exercise required for an effective warm-up will depend very much on a person's fitness level and the exercise to be performed in the main part of the workout. This is because changes in body temperature vary with body size, fat level and rate of body metabolism. In addition, sports differ tremendously in the demands they make on the body tissues, so a warm-up before a vigorous game of hockey would clearly need to be more extensive than one for a casual game of bowls. Equally, a top-level sprinter will require a more thorough warm-up session than a casual sportsman or woman, because the sprinter is likely to be able to push him or herself to a higher physical level. The following are guidelines:

- **Intensity**: If it is to be effective, a warm-up must be intense enough to cause mild sweating.

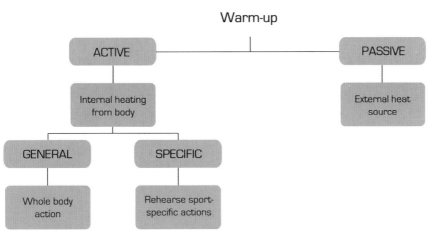

Figure 4.3 Types of warm-up

When this happens, it indicates that the inside (core) temperature of the body has increased by about 1°C. Increasing the core temperature by this amount has been shown to be the minimum requirement for bringing about the warm-up changes discussed above.

- **Clothing**: Because we are trying to raise the body temperature, it is best to perform the warm-up wearing warm clothing to keep the body heat in. The amount of clothing needed to provide adequate insulation will depend largely on the outside temperature. Light clothing may be suitable in a warm sports-hall, but thick fleecy material with a weatherproof covering layer will be needed on the touchline of a cold and windy pitch.

- **Activities**: Warm-up activities should be continuous and rhythmical in nature. Gentle jogging, light aerobics, or cycling on a static bicycle in the gym are all examples of good warm-up activities. Once light sweating has begun, the major joints should be taken through their full range of movement, starting with small movements which gradually become larger. Finally, some sport-specific actions must be included in the warm-up period as a part of skill rehearsal.

- **Time**: A good warm-up may take 10–15 minutes, but it is time well spent. Note that we are using a warm-up before stretching rather than using stretching as part of a warm-up. This makes sense because tissues will stretch more effectively when warm. The movements we use in the warm-up to take the major joints through their range of motion are not stretching exercises as such. The warm-up movements take the joints through their full range of motion, but do not try to increase this range of motion as stretching exercises would.

Key point:

Match your warm-up to your body requirements and exercise type and intensity.

WARM-DOWN

Just as it is vital to begin an exercise session slowly by warming up, so it is important to end it the same way by using a warm-down or cool-down. The warm-down period has a number of important effects.

First, during intense exercise the heartbeat increases, and the beating of the heart is actually helped by the contraction of the exercising limb muscles. As these muscles contract they squeeze the blood vessels that travel through them, thus helping the blood to return to the heart. If an individual stops exercising suddenly, the limb muscles no longer pump the blood vessels and help the heart. The demand placed on the heart is increased and the pulse will actually get faster even though exercise has stopped.

An effective warm-down can also reduce muscle ache. This is caused partly by lactic acid formation, and partly through tiny muscle tears that occur during very hard training. Hard training causes local swelling within a muscle, giving *delayed onset muscle soreness* (DOMS). In the case of DOMS, you feel fine the day after a workout, but the day after that you feel stiff. To reduce these effects you should perform a warm-down using similar exercises to those chosen for the warm-up, gradually lowering the exercise intensity until resting levels are reached. It is interesting to note that stretching exercises may be used to reduce muscle pain that occurs after intensive strength training.

Finally, shake your muscles to loosen and relax them, and take a warm shower to flush fresh blood through them and aid recovery. Because blood is still needed in the muscles after exercise in order to aid recovery, you should not eat a large meal immediately. If you feel hungry and in need of an 'energy boost' eat a small amount of sweet, high-carbohydrate food such as a banana or a piece of toast and honey.

Key point:

When planning your workout, allow at least 5 minutes for a warm-down. Do not fill all your time with hard exercise and then rush out of the gym.

OVERLOAD

To achieve a training effect, the body must be exposed to a physical stress that is greater than that encountered in everyday living. If this is done the body is said to be *overloaded*, and the body tissues will change or 'adapt' as a result, provided they are given time to do so. The two key points regarding overload are: that the overload must be greater than that normally encountered by the body; and that time is needed for the body tissues to adapt. Tissue adaptation of this type can be illustrated by something rubbing on the skin, such as a stone in a shoe. If the rubbing occurs continuously (without rest), the skin will break down and bleed. If, however, the rubbing occurs and then the skin is rested before being stressed again, a hard callus will form. In the former case, no recovery period was available for tissue adaptation, in the latter, tissue adaptation (callus growth) occurred in the recovery period itself. Exactly the same occurs with exercise.

If we take weight training as an example of this process, the resistance from the weight causes muscle breakdown. The body overcompensates by building stronger muscle in the rest period between exercise. For this reason, rest is vital, and intense exercise should not be practised every day, but on alternate days.

As fitness improves, exercise must become harder so the body continues to be taxed to the same degree. If the body has adapted to the training load, further improvement will only occur

Table 4.1	Overload components			
Type	**Frequency**	**Intensity**	**Time**	**Type**
F.I.T.T. component	How often?	How hard?	How long?	Which action?

if the training intensity is increased. Exercise must therefore be progressive (gradually getting harder) for the overload to have the same effect.

Overload has four components, summarised by the mnemonic FITT, standing for frequency, intensity, time, and type (*see* table 4.1).

- **Frequency**: The frequency must be appropriate – often enough for the tissues changes to build up, but not too often so that recovery is allowed.
- **Intensity**: Training must be intense enough to challenge the body tissues. The intensity of flexibility training may be assessed by the range of movement.
- **Time**: Training must be carried out for long enough for an overload to occur, but not so long that tissue damage results. The timing of a stretch is the holding time (static stretch), or ratio of movements (dynamic stretch).
- **Type**: The training type will dictate the tissue changes that will occur. The training is said to be 'specific' where the changes match the requirements of a particular sport. For each of the components of fitness (*see* table 4.2) a different training type is required. When training for stamina the intensity of exercise may be determined by the pulse rate, and when training for strength by the weight lifted.

The American College of Sports Medicine (ACSM) defined the appropriate overload for health-related exercise in 1978, and this was updated in 1990 and again in 2002, and is regularly updated to take on research findings. They say that the quality and quantity of exercise required to maintain aerobic fitness and body composition is a training frequency of three to five days per week at an intensity of between 60–90 per cent of the age-related maximal heart rate. This should be carried out for 20–60 minutes each time and be rhythmical or continuous in nature. Resistance training should be performed for one set of 8–12 repetitions of 8–10 exercises for the major muscle groups for two days per week, and involve both machine and free weight exercise.

From the point of view of stretching, the ACSM says: Flexibility exercises should be incorporated into the overall fitness programme sufficient to develop and maintain range of motion (ROM). These exercises should stretch the major muscle groups and be performed a minimum of 2–3 days a week. Stretching should include appropriate static and/or dynamic techniques … Static stretches should be held for 10–30 seconds … PNF techniques should include a 6 second contraction followed by a 10–30-second assisted stretch. So, their general advice is to stretch on a regular basis and hold the stretches for longer than has traditionally been recommended in sport. In addition, the effects of a warm-up make it desirable to perform a warm-up before stretching if the aim is to improve range of motion (developmental stretching). However, if the aim is simply to maintain the range of motion (maintenance stretching), the stretches themselves may form part of the warm-up or exercise programme.

Key point:

General guidelines for stretching are to: (a) stretch the major joints and two-joint muscles 3–5 times per week; (b) hold each stretch for 20–30 seconds; and (c) stretch after a warm-up of sufficient intensity to induce light sweating.

Table 4.2	Fitness components ('S' factor)
Stamina	Cardiopulmonary and local muscle endurance
Suppleness	Active, passive, PNF
Strength	Concentric, eccentric, isometric
Speed	Speed (rate of movement), power (rate of doing work)
Skill	Balance and coordination
Specificity	Exercise must match required training outcome
Spirit	Psychological factors of training

TRAINING EFFECTS

We have seen that an overload on body tissue gives a training effect. This effect is largely reversible, however. If training stops, the benefits achieved for each fitness component will be lost and 'detraining' will occur.

In just 20 days of total rest, stamina reduces by 25 per cent – a loss of about 1 per cent per day. Strength reduction is even greater, with average losses over the same period of 35 per cent. Muscles that have become more flexible with training will slowly tighten again, and muscle imbalance may occur if some muscles tighten more quickly than others (see page 69). Skill-based components including sports technique, balance and coordination last longer, but will gradually degrade with time. The principle is clear – 'use it or lose it!'

Training has immediate, short-term and long-term effects:

- Immediate effects are the body's responses to exercise. These are brought about by increased metabolism and include higher heart and breathing rates, changes in blood flow, increased body temperature, and chemical alterations to enzymes within the working muscles.

- Short-term training effects become apparent when exercise stops and the body tries to reduce its metabolic rate to resting levels once more. Body temperature has increased, so sweating continues to try to cool the tissues. Energy has been used and must be replaced, so breathing rate and heart rate remain high. Waste products have been formed as energy was 'burnt', and these wastes must be eliminated.

- Long-term effects are the cumulative results of exercise, reflecting the body's adaptation to training. Intense training stresses the body; over time, the body learns from this and changes so that the next training bout will not stress it as much. If a training session is not intense enough, it will not stress the body sufficiently and no adaptation will occur. However, if it is too intense and the body cannot cope, injury may result. Following training, time must be allowed for the body to change and adapt; rest for recovery from exercise is vital.

COMPONENTS OF FITNESS

It is generally accepted that two types of fitness exist: health-related and task- (performance) related. These include various components which can be described as 'S' factors for convenience (see table 4.2). Health-related fitness includes components that are considered to be beneficial to health. In this context the term *stamina* is used to encompass both heart-lung fitness and muscle endurance. This fitness component is important to the health of the heart and circulatory system. *Suppleness* (flexibility) and *strength* are concerned with the health of the musculo-skeletal system, and are important in injury prevention.

These three components are all essential to sports performance, but in addition *speed* and *skilled action* are required. Speed involves rapid muscle contraction and the elastic abilities of the muscle and is important for explosive events.

Skill includes the skills needed for a particular sport, as well as general physical skills such as balance and coordination.

Injury will be more likely if the fitness components become unbalanced. For example, an inexperienced bodybuilder may have excessive strength in comparison with their flexibility, making muscle pulls more likely. A poorly trained distance runner may have a lot of stamina to protect the heart, but very little strength or flexibility, leaving the joints open to injury. Many keep-fit enthusiasts see themselves as 'very fit' because they may be strong and supple and have plenty of stamina, but endless hours spent working on gym machines will do little to improve skill, and fitness enthusiasts can be left clumsy with poor balance and coordination ability. So the message is clear: an overall training programme must work on all the fitness components if it is to be totally effective.

SPECIFICITY

Over a period of time, the demands placed on the body during exercise cause the body to change. With stretching, the muscles become more flexible; with weight training they become stronger; and with running, stamina improves. These changes are the adaptations to exercise and will closely match the type of demand placed on the body. For example, running marathons will improve aerobic endurance, while sprinting will build anaerobic power. If we wanted to improve our distance running ability there would be little point in using sprint training, because the body adaptation that would occur would not be the right one.

SAID PRINCIPLE

The above example illustrates an important principle, that of *training specificity*. We can say that all training follows the SAID principle: 'specific adaptation to imposed demand'. Put simply, this dictates that the change that takes place in the body (the adaptation) will closely resemble (be specific to) the type of training used (the imposed demand).

Applying this principle to stretching means that, when choosing stretching exercises to improve sports performance, we must match the range of motion, the muscles stretched, and the muscle balance around a joint to similar actions in the desired sport. For example, if a soccer player needs stretching exercises, these can be designed for the muscles used in kicking. The exercises should take account of any tightness a player may already have, and the stretching programme should be individually designed. Also, stretching should be applied as part of a general training programme, so that increases in flexibility are matched by strength improvements, which enable the player to control the new range of motion that he or she has gained.

FLEXIBILITY TRAINING

WHAT STOPS A JOINT MOVING THROUGH AN INFINITE RANGE OF MOTION?

We need to look at two areas to explain this: internal (body) factors and external (environmental) factors.

One important internal factor is bone. Obviously, we cannot affect the amount of bone in a joint, but we must be aware of it as a limiting factor to flexibility. After a fracture, for example, the amount of bone will increase over the fracture site. If this area is near a joint, range of motion may be reduced: in this case it would be fruitless to continue a stretching programme to this region. Equally, an elderly athlete may have osteoarthrosis, a condition in which the bone surfaces of the joints become uneven and more bone is formed. Again, the bone itself may limit movement and it would be dangerous to attempt any forceful stretching manoeuvres. Soft tissues such as tendons, ligaments, the joint capsule and the skin itself will limit movement. These tissues are *inert*, i.e. they do not contract. However, they do have elastic properties so they will stretch. Muscle is also an important factor: it is contractile and its contraction is governed by a number of important reflexes. Surrounding the muscle, however, is a connective tissue framework that will limit movement, so a muscle may be seen as both an inert and contractile structure.

The most important external factor that affects flexibility is temperature. When warmed, the body tissues become more pliable. A thorough warm-up must, therefore, be performed before stretching exercises are attempted. Often, vigorous stretching exercises are performed as a warm-up, which is incorrect: until the tissues are warm, and an athlete starts to sweat lightly, full-range stretching exercises should not be attempted. In the same way that warm tissue is more pliable, cold tissue is stiffer. Research has shown that when stretching is used after injury, a greater range of motion can be achieved if the muscle is cooled with ice while holding it in its final stretched position.

INDIVIDUAL DIFFERENCES IN FLEXIBILITY

If you ask the members of any class to perform a stretching exercise, you immediately see a tremendous variation in movement: some will be more flexible than others; some will move into the position in a smooth and effortless way; while others will stumble clumsily into the exercise. The differences reflect variations in both range of movement and skill-level between individuals.

People involved in strength and power events are usually less flexible than those who use their own bodyweight as resistance, such as swimmers, gymnasts and dancers. The degree of flexibility depends also on whether a person's fitness programme is balanced. Inexperienced bodybuilders who just train for strength and bulk are among the least flexible, while teenage girl gymnasts can be among the most flexible.

Females are generally more flexible than males, especially around the hip and shoulder. Hormonal changes will also affect flexibility in females. During pregnancy, and to a lesser extent during menstruation, *relaxin* hormone is released into the bloodstream. This, together with progesterone and oestrogen, has the effect of relaxing the pelvic ligaments, and making the joint between the base of the spine and the pelvis (the sacroiliac joint) more mobile. The effects of hormone changes may remain for as long as six months after pregnancy, so during this time the person is at risk from rapid end-range stretching exercises.

Range of movement is also dictated by lifestyle and previous injury. Inactive individuals who get the exercise message late in life will be inflexible, and in many cases the range of movement they gain will never be as great as the range they could have achieved had they been active all their lives. In addition, the limitation to range of movement can often be permanent, dictated by years of poor posture and faulty movement techniques. Previous injuries can leave a reduced range of movement as the only outward sign that problems have occurred. People with a history of low back pain will often be tight in the lower spine and hamstring muscles, while those with shoulder problems may be left with limited shoulder rotation movements. In cases where an individual's flexibility is asymmetrical (greater on one side of the body than the other), a flexibility programme must aim to restore symmetry and not just increase range of movement.

FLEXIBILITY AND BODY TYPE

Each of us has a different type of body: some are fatter, some are thinner, and some are more or less muscled. The degree to which we differ can be partially explained by our 'body type' or *somatotype*. Three extreme body types are recognised: *mesomorphs* (muscular); *endomorphs* (fatter); and *ectomorphs* (thinner) (*see* fig 4.4).

- Mesomorphs have more bone and muscle development. Their bodies are made for strenuous physical activity, and individuals of this type tend to be heavily muscled. The chest is broad, and the shoulders are wider than the waist – the 'Tarzan' type.
- Endomorphs have rounder physiques and they tend to put on and store fat. They have a 'pear drop' appearance with the abdomen being as large, or larger than the chest – the typical 'Billy Bunter' character.
- Ectomorphs have long delicate limbs – the traditional 'bean-poles'.

In reality, few people have physiques that fall firmly into just one of these categories. We are all a mixture of the three extremes. By taking height, weight, bone size, limb girth and body-fat measurements, an individual can be given a score indicating the proportion of each body-type component present in their physiques.

Scores range from one to seven, and are presented in the order endomorph/mesomorph/ectomorph. Thus a highly endomorphic individual would score 7/1/1 and a high mesomorph 1/7/1. The somatotype rating can be illustrated graphically so that somatotype averages for different sports can be compared (*see* fig 4.5). We can see, for example, that both gymnasts and basketball players have a high degree of mesomorphy, but that the basketball players have a greater tendency to endomorphy than do the gymnasts. Bodybuilders are highly mesomorphic, as we would expect. Both ballet dancers and swimmers are roughly average on all scores, possibly reflecting the fact that these athletes use their own bodyweight as resistance.

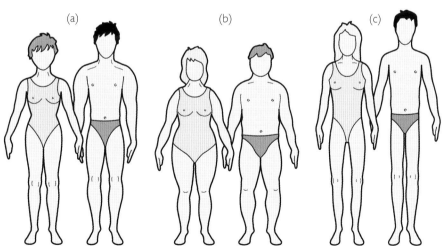

Figure 4.4 Somatotypes – the three extremes of body types (a) mesomorphs, (b) endomorphs and (c) ectomorphs

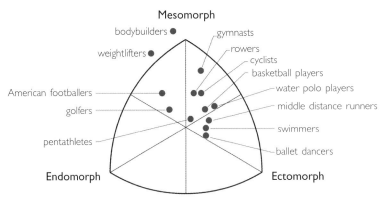

Figure 4.5 Elite athlete somatotypes

PHYSIOLOGICAL EFFECTS OF STRETCHING EXERCISE

Most people would recognise that stretching exercises make you more flexible. In other words, you are able to stretch further because your range of motion is greater. In addition, it is a common observation that with stretching, movements seem somehow easier to perform. What are the mechanisms that achieve these changes?

Habituation

One of the first changes to occur in stretching is an alteration in the stretch reflex. When a muscle is stretched rapidly, its tone increases as a result of the stretch reflex. This is a protective mechanism designed partly to prevent the muscle from getting injured if it is pulled suddenly, but, more importantly, it is part of a postural mechanism called a saving reaction. Because we stand on two feet rather than four, our base of support is very small compared to our height. If you consider a closed-up step ladder, it balances on two feet and is about 5 or 6 feet tall. This is similar to a human. Place the step ladder on its end, however, and it will fall over; not so with the human. The reason that we do not fall is, for the main part, due to the stretch reflex. As we begin to topple forwards, our feet are pushed

into dorsiflexion at the ankle and our calf muscles stretched. A stretch reflex occurs in these muscles and they contract to press the toes into the floor and prevent us from falling. As the toes press into the floor, we begin to fall backwards, but once again a stretch reflex occurs to prevent this. At any one time, dozens of stretch reflexes are taking place to stop us from falling and we sway backwards, forwards and side-to-side in a constant battle with gravity. This continuous movement is called postural sway.

So, the stretch reflex is a protective mechanism that increases muscle tone. When we are performing stretching exercises, however, we can override this to actually reduce muscle tone. If we stretch the muscle over and over again, eventually the reflex becomes dulled or 'desensitised' and will not respond to the stretch to the same extent. The process of desensitising the stretch reflex in this way is called *habituation*. It requires repeated stimulation with the same stimulus to improve; in other words, the stretch must be rhythmical (pulsing) rather than haphazard.

The point at which the stretch reflex occurs is known as the 'threshold' (*see* fig 4.6). The threshold is higher after repeated stretching, meaning that the muscle can be stretched to a greater range before the stretch reflex occurs.

Definition:

Habituation is the reduction and eventual loss of a response or sensation as a result of continuous stimulation with a constant stimulus.

Stiffness changes

When a muscle is stretched, it will pull back using *elastic recoil*. This is the same as for any substance: for example, if we stretch an elastic band it will recoil. Similarly, if we try to stretch a piece of string it will also recoil, but to a lesser extent than the elastic band. This is because the string is less elastic than the band, and therefore more rigid, or stiffer. Because it is stiffer, the string offers more resistance to the stretching movement than the elastic band. To make the string stretch further, we would have to reduce its stiffness and, in so doing, its resistance to motion. This process is exactly what happens with muscle. When a muscle is stretched, it resists the stretch because it has a certain stiffness, which is somewhere between the elastic band and the string. With repeated stretching, however, its stiffness reduces. The process that is occurring here is a little like warming putty.

Stretch putty and it is quite stiff; hold it in your hands and it becomes warm and less stiff, enabling you to stretch it more easily. The same is true of muscle. If you perform a warm-up, the warming of the tissues makes the muscles less stiff and so easier to stretch. Simply by performing a stretching exercise, the same will happen due to the changes in muscle tone that occur. In fact, the stiffness reduction that occurs after a 10 minute period of jogging as a warm-up is exactly the same as that which occurs after 5 repetitions of a static stretch, holding each repetition for 30 seconds. The reduction in stiffness is about

Time

Point at which stretch reflex occurs – 'threshold'

[A]

Higher threshold level [A] means stretch reflex occurs later in movement range

Figure 4.6 Habituation of the stretch reflex during stretch exercise

4–5 per cent following this type of stretching; this may not seem much, but if you imagine the number of steps an athlete takes when running a marathon, for example, you can see that a 5 per cent reduction in stiffness will use less energy and may even reduce the likelihood of injury.

Key point:

With stretching, a muscle becomes less stiff and offers less resistance to movement.

Stretch tolerance

We have seen that muscle flexibility can alter due to muscle stiffness changes. However, at the start of a stretching programme the first changes we see can be independent of alteration in the electrical signals (EMG) coming from the muscle. It seems that the immediate effect of the stretch is an alteration in the amount of discomfort the user is willing to tolerate, or their *stretch tolerance*. The sensation of putting a stretch on a muscle is very intense and, to someone not used to training, this can be interpreted as potentially damaging to the muscle. Feedback systems tend to protect the body from harm, and so any stimulus that is interpreted as a threat will result in a subconscious unwillingness to allow the movement to occur. As the pain of the stretch becomes more familiar, rather than being interpreted negatively as a threat, the pain is interpreted positively as a function of training. The person is therefore more willing to tolerate a greater level of stretch and the resulting greater discomfort; in other words, the individual experiences less pain for the same amount of stretch.

Key point:

Stretching causes muscle pain, but over time there is a pain-relieving effect and more stretching can be tolerated.

Changes in muscle sarcomeres

Both changes in muscle tone and muscle stiffness are called *acute* changes, as they occur after relatively short periods of training (months). However, after many years of training, long-term or *chronic* changes may occur. We saw on pages 31–32 that muscles contract by using sliding filaments, and that a unit or block of these sliding filaments taken together is called a sarcomere. As a muscle is contracted, the filaments of the muscle slide together and the sarcomere gets shorter. As the muscle relaxes and is stretched, the filaments move apart and the sarcomere gets longer. This occurs in each sarcomere in the chain right through the length of the muscle. Over a period of time, repeatedly stretching the sarcomeres causes the muscle to adapt by increasing the number of sacromeres in each of the chains. Because the sarcomeres are lined up one after another (in a series), we call this an increase in *serial sarcomere number* (SSN). This

is more commonly seen in individuals who have practised a sport where stretching is an integral part of training, such as ballet.

Key point:

Over very long periods, muscle can adapt by actually growing longer.

FLEXIBILITY METHODS

We have seen that range of motion can be limited by both inert structures and by the contractile portion of the muscle. Muscle reflexes are important when trying to stretch muscles, while an adequate warm-up is needed to make the tissues more pliable before we stretch. Following a warm-up, the body should be kept warm throughout the stretching period by using warm, loose-fitting clothing such as jogging bottoms and a sweatshirt.

Stretches may be *static*, where no movement is involved, *dynamic*, where the limb is moved as it is stretched, or use **proprioceptive neuromuscular facilitation (PNF)** stretching, a muscle reflex-based technique.

These basic types have a number of sub-divisions (*see* table 4.3). Pulsing is an extension of static stretching, active and ballistic are both dynamic movements performed at different speeds, and contract–relax (CR) or CRAC are PNF techniques. The flexibility types are compared in terms of safety, ease of application, effectiveness and time to apply in figure 4.7.

Key point:

The three major categories of stretches are static, dynamic and PNF.

Type	Safety	Ease of application	Effectiveness	Time to apply
Static	****	*****	***	****
pulsing	**	***	****	****
Dynamic	***	****	*****	**
active	*****	***	****	*****
ballistic	*	***	**	**
PNF				
CR	****	**	****	**
CRAC	****	*	*****	*

Figure 4.7 Comparison of stretching techniques

Static stretching

Static stretching involves taking a limb to the point at which tightness is felt and holding this position. This is the sort of flexibility used in yoga, for example. As the position is held, the inert structures gradually elongate, while the muscle reflexes detect tension in the muscle tendon and gradually allow the muscle to relax. This is a particularly safe method of stretching, but because the position is held for up to 30 seconds the starting position chosen for the exercise must be comfortable and well supported. Lying and sitting on a mat are good starting positions, but kneeling and single leg standing are not. Once the position is achieved, concentration on breathing out and 'sighing' can allow the muscle to relax further. When the stretch is released, the muscle tension must come off slowly without allowing the tissues to 'spring' back.

Static stretching should generally be applied for 4–5 repetitions, with each stretch being released and the limb rested for 10–20 seconds before the next rep is used. With each rep the range of motion should be seen to gradually improve.

Table 4.3	Stretching types	
STATIC	**DYNAMIC**	**PNF**
Hold	Active	Contract relax
Pulsing	Ballistic	CRAC

Pulsing

Static stretching is sometimes used with small presses at the end of the range of movement (really moving it into the dynamic category). This is termed *pulsing*, and involves little more than tensing the tissue then releasing it, and repeating this action rhythmically. The repetition causes the muscle reflexes to become accustomed to the stretch and they desensitise (or habituate) to the movement. This process occurs when the body simply gets used to a repeated stimulus and no longer reacts to it. Although this occurs in both ballistic stretching and pulsing, the smaller movements used in pulsing greatly reduce the momentum built up and so the potential for injury is much lower. The downside of pulsing is that it may not match the high-speed, through-range acceleration used in a particular sport, and so does not provide training specifically for a ballistic sport such as martial arts, for example. It can, however, be built into a programme to greatly reduce the amount of time spent purely on ballistic movement.

Dynamic stretching

Many stretching exercises are used in isolation from other actions and at slow speed. This enables the user to accurately target a particular muscle and is also the best way of avoiding injury, especially for inexperienced exercisers or those returning to stretching after a torn muscle, for example. However, this isolation takes the single muscle action out of the full motor programme of a particular movement. Each movement in sport consists of a number of actions joined together in a chain of movement called a *motor programme*. For example, a jump creates movement (and therefore stretch) at the ankle, knee, hip, trunk and arm. If we simply stretch the calf and Achilles, we will increase the flexibility of this region, but only in isolation from the other body parts and at a speed that fails to match that of the jump action in sport. We could therefore say that slow controlled stretching – although potentially safe and easy to learn – is not truly functional. In other words, using this type of training in isolation will enhance the specific muscle stretch but not the movement performance. This is where dynamic stretching comes in.

Dynamic stretching is, literally, stretching with movement. A dynamic stretch is a controlled movement through the full range of motion at either single or multiple joints. Essentially, it involves placing the stretch within the context of a functional action, whether for a specific sport or for daily activities such as lifting. The advantage is that it involves stretching, muscle contraction, muscle control and movement rehearsal (skill and timing). For example, a dynamic stretch for jumping would be practised at a speed between that of a static stretch (no movement) and that of a full jump (rapid movement). The speed of the movement and the complexity of its action are introduced progressively (*see* fig 4.8) until the action is eventually practised at full functional speed. At this point, a dynamic stretch has often progressed to full plyometric training (*see* page 37). A comparison of some of the features of static and dynamic stretching is shown in table 4.4.

Active stretching

Active stretching is a slower-speed version of classic dynamic stretching. It involves an active contraction (isometric or concentric) of one muscle to its full inner range, requiring the antagonist to stretch fully to its outer range. Active stretching tends to be used as part of a muscle imbalance correction programme and so is *clinically* based, while dynamic stretching is generally used for fitness and sport and so is *performance* based.

Ballistic stretching

Ballistic stretching is similar to dynamic stretching, but is performed at very high speeds and generally to repetition. Two factors are important here. First, when the whole body or trunk is used, the weight of the body moving at speed will build up *momentum*. The energy contained within the momentum can make it impossible to stop the movement soon enough, so tissues can be overstretched and repeated small tears called microtrauma can occur. Over the years this can cause a build-up of scar tissue, altering the mechanics of a joint. Second, the stretch reflex dictates that a rapid stretch will cause muscles to subsequently contract and tighten. Instead of increasing range of motion, the range may then actually reduce. It becomes obvious that this type of stretching can be both dangerous and ineffective in many situations.

However, ballistic stretching can have an important role when carried out under the supervision of a physiotherapist after injury. The reason is that many sports, such as the martial arts, actually involve full-range actions and a high degree of flexibility. If the actions are performed slowly they are dynamic flexibility actions, but when performed explosively – as they often are competitively – they become ballistic actions. The athlete practising this sport does not get injured each time he kicks, simply because he has trained his body to reset the stretch reflex so that it does not occur at the speed at which he is kicking.

If the athlete should suffer an injury, however, he must regain lost strength and flexibility and

Static stretch of calf/Achilles and rectus femoris

↓

Static stretch of calf/Achilles combined with rectus femoris

↓

Dynamic slow-speed stretch from half-squat position to full standing

↓

Dynamic mid-/half-speed stretch, as above

↓

Dynamic slow-speed stretch from full-squat position to full standing

↓

Dynamic slow-speed stretch, as above, with small jump

↓

Dynamic fast-speed stretch with larger jump

↓

Full plyometric action to repetition

Figure 4.8 Example of progression of a dynamic stretching for jumping

gradually reintroduce ballistic flexibility before attempting competitive sport once more. This must be done in a highly controlled and supervised manner. Initially, only mid-range movements are used, then gradually the range of motion is increased over many training sessions. It must be emphasised that full static, active and PNF flexibility, and full strength and power, should be regained before any ballistic actions are used. The danger comes when inexperienced athletes try to copy a person who has been training with this type of action for many years. The body of the inexperienced athlete has not had time to adapt itself to these highly specialised actions, so injury is the frequent outcome.

PNF stretching

PNF (proprioceptive neuromuscular facilitation) stretching is a method adapted from physiotherapy treatment of patients who have had strokes. It involves a series of movements designed to get the maximum out of a muscle by using primitive muscle reflexes.

Contract–relax

The first PNF technique is called *contract–relax* (CR). With this method, the athlete must first contract the muscle to be stretched and hold the contraction for 10–20 seconds. During this period the golgi tendon organs will register the tension build-up and cause autogenic inhibition, allowing an increased range of motion to be achieved. Because the muscle is tensed isometrically, this technique is also called *post-isometric relaxation* (PIR) and is also used as part of *muscle energy technique* (MET).

Contract–relax–agonist–contract

The second PNF technique is called *contract–relax–agonist–contract* (CRAC). This consists of the contract–relax method first, but goes further by using the fact that when one muscle contracts, its opposing neighbour (the antagonist) must relax. This reflex, called *reciprocal innervation* (*see* page 34), allows us to stretch still further. To perform the CRAC method, the muscle to be stretched is first contracted and held for 20 seconds. This muscle is then relaxed, a brief pause is allowed, and then the opposing muscle is contracted to pull further into the stretched position. This has the added benefit of strengthening the muscle group that controls the range of motion, but can be difficult for some individuals to correctly practise unsupervised.

General stretching guidelines are summarised in table 4.6.

STARTING POSITIONS

The starting position for any stretching exercise is important both in terms of safety and effectiveness. It must allow free movement of the part of the body that is to be stretched, and it must be stable. An unstable position can cause a person to lose balance and, therefore, lose control of a movement, placing excessive strain on the tissues being stretched. In addition, positions that are uncomfortable do not allow individuals to relax completely, and excessive tension in a muscle is not conducive to effective stretching. Furthermore, some individuals with medical conditions will find that certain starting positions, which place excessive or unbalanced stress on a weakened part of the body, are unsuitable. Table 4.5 shows a variety of common starting positions with points to note and suggested modifications.

USE OF APPARATUS

Any form of training requires the body to be overloaded sufficiently to cause an adaptation. In the case of stretching exercises, the overload is to increase the range of motion and hold the position. This is normally achieved manually, but apparatus may be used. Most commonly, a towel or belt is used to support the part of the body being stretched and to allow greater relaxation. For example, when a subject is quite inflexible, thigh stretches are sometimes easier if a towel is placed around the foot. Belts and pads may be used to keep the spine straight when hip exercises are used, as there is a tendency to allow the spine to round, increasing lumbar stress.

Various machines are available to facilitate adductor stretches in the hope of achieving the classic 'splits' position. These are normally hydraulic or ratchet devices that force the legs further into abduction. From the point of view of safety, the amount of force used and its point of application are of paramount importance.

Forcing the hips into an abducted position can place an excessive stress on the hip tissues. Applying this force below the knee can stress the medial ligament of the knee by imposing an inward (valgus) stress on these structures.

Table 4.4	Comparison of static and dynamic stretching
Static	**Dynamic**
• Isolates body part	• Uses several body parts simultaneously
• Able to focus on single structure	• Faster action
• Slow and controlled	• Involves several fitness components
• Uses single fitness component	• Can be used to match functional movement
• Starting position usually fully supported	• Movement rehearsal
• Little skill required	• Skill and timing used

Table 4.5	Starting positions for stretching exercises	
Starting position	**Points to note**	**Modifications**
Standing	Individuals must stand in an erect and balanced posture. Common errors are to stand in a slumped or round-shouldered posture which does not allow correct spinal movement. With the feet together the position is unstable, especially if an individual has poor balance. The bodyweight must be taken equally through both legs.	Standing with feet apart (stride standing), or with one foot in front of the other (walk standing), facing the direction of movement. Improve stability further by holding on to an object (support standing).
Walk standing (one foot in front of the other) Step standing (one foot up on a step)	Both positions are more stable than standing alone, but excessive stress may be placed on the knee if leg alignment is not correct. Ensure that the knee passes directly over the middle of the foot on the leading leg.	Use the thigh of the leading leg to lean on for support.
Supine lying	If the hip flexors are tight the pelvis may be tilted forwards, increasing the lumbar lordosis and placing pressure on the lumbar spine (see page 74). In individuals who have little body fat and prominent pubic bones, pressure from a hard floor on body prominences can be painful. Some elderly subjects find lying makes breathing difficult for them, and some with arthritis of the neck joints find lying without a pillow causes dizziness and nausea.	Always lie on a padded mat. Use a rolled towel beneath the lower spine for support. Elderly people might find it more comfortable to raise their necks on a small pillow or folded towel. Bend the knees (crook lying) to relax the hip flexors and reduce pressure on the lumbar spine.
Prone lying	Individuals must turn the head to one side to be able to breathe freely, and this can place excessive stress on the neck if the position is held. Pressure over prominent pelvic bones can be painful, and male subjects may find testicular compression occurs. Those with patellar pain find compression on a hard surface extremely painful.	Always use a well-padded mat, and encourage male subjects to press testicles away from compression from the pubic bone. Place a rolled towel below the forehead to enable the subject to breathe freely without compressing the nose. Bend the knees and place a rolled towel beneath the ankles.
Sitting	When the hips are flexed further than 45 degrees, tightness in the hip tissues begins to tilt the pelvis and flatten the spine. Eventually the spine may round, giving back pain after prolonged periods. Holding the head too far forwards places stress on the neck and shoulder muscles.	Encourage individuals to 'sit tall' and avoid slumping. Sit with knees apart to allow the pelvis to tilt freely and maintain the lumbar lordosis.
Kneeling	Pressure on the front of the knee is very painful. Kneeling on all fours (prone kneeling) may place stress on the wrist. Kneeling on the knees only (high kneeling) places increased stress on the patella and can be unstable.	Use a well-padded mat. Ensure that the knees are shoulder width apart to aid stability. Hold on to an object when using high kneeling.

Table 4.6	Stretching guidelines
Stretching type	**Technique**
Static	• Take limb to end of range • Hold for 20–30 seconds
Pulsing	• Take limb to end of range and stop • Perform 10–20 small amplitude (2–3 cm) presses
Dynamic	• Take limb through full range of motion combining several movement planes e.g. flexion/abduction/rotation) • Mimic sports actions
Active	• Take limb to end of range by contracting opposite muscle maximally • Use to correct muscle imbalance
Ballistic	• Perform repeated vigorous full-range action used in sport • Practise at competition speed
CR	• Contract muscle to be stretched against partner-applied resistance • Relax, and then apply static stretch using partner to guide limb
CRAC	• Contract muscle to be stretched against partner resistance • Relax, and then pull limb into stretched position using opposite muscle • Final force supplied by user

Continuous passive motion (CPM) machines have been used in a hospital setting for a number of years, and these are now being seen in the sporting context. The machines are electrically powered, and move the joints through a specified range for a set period. The amount of force available makes it essential that these machines are used only under the direct supervision of a qualified physiotherapist.

Stretching frames are also common. These enable the user to take up a more stable body position and reduce the likelihood of 'wobbling' and potentially falling. Some are simply modifications of the traditional wall bar found in school gyms, while others enable the user to sit and perform a variety of stretches from the sitting position as well as from standing.

DEVELOPING AGILITY

We have seen that fitness is composed of a number of components. Of these, flexibility – the ability to obtain a range of motion about a joint – is only one. Agility, by comparison, is the ability to use and control this range of motion. For this reason, good agility requires a number of fitness components: flexibility, strength, muscle endurance, skill, and speed. Agility is thus fundamental to good sports performance.

Agility exercises involve using controlled movements through a full range of motion, and may be used individually or in a circuit training format. Examples include movements from dance, ballet, aerobics and gymnastics, together with sport-specific actions requiring a high degree of agility.

SUMMARY

- Warming up has been shown to lessen the number of irregular heartbeats and reduce the blood pressure during exercise. It will also make tissue more pliable and will affect psychological arousal.
- During a warm-up the movements to be practised during a workout should be rehearsed.
- Both active (exercise) and passive (heating) warm-ups may be used.
- When the body is exposed to a physical stress greater than the stress experienced in normal everyday activities, it is said to be overloaded.
- In 20 days' total rest stamina reduces by 25 per cent and strength by 35 per cent.
- Training specificity means that the change that takes place in the body as a result of exercise will closely match the type of exercise that is used.
- Stretching achieves its effects by changing muscle reflexes, making muscle less stiff and relieving the pain of the stretch.
- Long-term effects of stretching can make a muscle grow longer.
- Three body types exist: mesomorph (muscular), endomorph (fatter) and ectomorph (thinner).
- We are all a mixture of these three types.
- Stretching may be static, dynamic or PNF.

5

// POSTURE

WHY IS POSTURE IMPORTANT?

Posture is simply the relationship (alignment) between different parts of the body. Posture is important from two standpoints. First, good posture underlies all exercise techniques. Exercises started from a basis of poor posture tend to be awkward and clumsy, with unequal tension placed on some body tissues. This can eventually lead to the accumulation of stress and consequent overuse injuries. Second, postural stress in daily life overworks some tissues and underworks others, leading to an imbalance of flexibility and strength. In the short term this imbalance gives rise to postural pain; but in the long term, because joints are pulled out of alignment, altered joint mechanics can lead to the development of joint surface degeneration (*see* fig 5.1 (c)).

Posture is maintained by both muscles and non-contractile tissues. A good posture is one in which the different parts of the body are correctly aligned, thus placing the minimum amount of stress on the body tissues. A good posture requires little muscle activity, so it is more relaxed and needs less energy to maintain it. At the same time, joint structures are not overstretched or shortened so much that they cause strain. In both of these cases, a good posture is one that is balanced. It therefore follows that a poor posture requires greater muscle work to maintain it and will almost certainly result in muscle fatigue. In addition, the increased joint-loading forces that result from poor posture increase the likelihood of pain and possible injury.

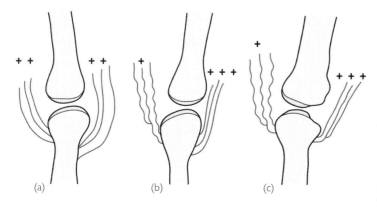

Figure 5.1 Muscle imbalance altering joint mechanics: (a) symmetrical muscle tone – normal joint; (b) unequal muscle pull (imbalance) – joint alignment poor; (c) joint surface degeneration

Two types of posture are important. Static posture is that seen at rest, while dynamic posture is that of motion – the type of body position a person takes up when moving. Static posture may be assessed by close inspection of the body, but the study of dynamic posture requires more in-depth training, and often the use of advanced laboratory facilities.

A number of factors interact to create a person's static posture. Body type and genetic make-up are important, as are strength and flexibility. In addition, the way a person sees themselves (their body image) and the mental state of an individual will affect their posture.

An individual cannot easily alter their genetic make-up, so the posture with which they were genetically endowed is largely permanent unless surgically changed. Children, for example, who have particular spinal deformities often require a number of complex operations to straighten the spine. Similarly, bone or skeletal 'frame size' is constant for an individual, so a stretching programme must take this into account.

The important factor in the development of both flexibility and strength is symmetry. An unequal development of either of these two elements can pull the body out of alignment, causing postural faults.

The balance between postural muscles and movement muscles is also important. Postural muscles hold us up against gravity and include those trunk muscles that give us 'core stability'. Movement muscles will create great power and

are able to move rapidly, but will tend to tighten. The combination of tightness (too much tone) of some muscles and sagging (too little tone) of other muscles results in muscle imbalance, which changes our postural alignment and gives rise to postural pain.

ASSESSING STANDING POSTURE

FROM BEHIND

When the body is viewed from behind, with the feet three inches apart, a vertical line should divide it into two equal halves. The pelvic rims (anterior superior iliac spines) should be in the same horizontal plane, and the pubis and pelvic rims should be in the same vertical plane. An individual's posture can be assessed by comparison with a score chart (*see* table 5.1). Anatomical 'landmarks' are compared with horizontal levels on the right and left sides of the body and include: the knee creases, buttock creases, pelvic rim, angle of the shoulder blades, upper arm bones, ears and skull protuberances. In addition, the alignment of the spinous processes and rib angles is observed. The distance between the arms and the trunk (keyhole), skin creases and unequal muscle bulk are indicators of asymmetrical posture. Slight side bending of the spine (scoliosis) becomes more noticeable when a person bends forwards (Adam's position) and a marked hump is seen over the twisted ribs.

Table 5.1	Assessment of standing position from behind		
	Ear level – hair line		Skin creases
	Shoulder level – cervical spine		Levels of pelvic rim, asis, belt line
	Inferior angle of scapula		Buttock creases
	Overall spinal alignment		Knee creases Muscle bulk
	Keyhole		Mid-line Achilles angle
	Adam's position		Foot position

Looking closely at the shoulder blade (scapula), the inner edge of the blade should be vertical and no more than three finger breadths from the spine. The blade should appear flat against the ribcage, and no part of it should jut out or appear prominent. The appearance of the shoulder area on the right and left sides of the body should be roughly the same (symmetrical). The bulk of the muscles around the shoulder should be even, with no one area appearing either 'muscle-bound' (excessive bulging) or 'wasted' (hollow). Finally, the contour of the muscle between the shoulder and neck (the upper fibres of the trapezius) should be smooth and rounded, rather than straight and tight like a cord.

FROM THE SIDE

From the side a vertical line (posture line) should pass just in front of the ankle bone (lateral

Key point:

When looking at a person's posture from behind, symmetry is important. Are both sides more or less equal?

malleolus), just in front of the centre of the knee joint, through the greater trochanter of the hip, then the bodies of the lumbar vertebrae and the centre of the shoulder joint and ear (*see* fig 5.3).

Because the posture line passes through the knee joint centre, the knee is pressed straight and locks (extensor torque), meaning that you do not require any muscle activity in your quadriceps to stay standing upright. If the knee moves forwards, the line passes behind the knee centre giving the knee a tendency to bend and unlock (flexor torque) this action must be resisted by activity in the quads. This muscle activity has two effects; first it is tiring over time. Second the patella is pressed on to the patellar surface of the femur below. For someone with patellofemoral pain this can worsen their condition.

Also compare the knee alignment for both sides, go round to the other side of your client to do this. The ankle, knee and hip should be in line. It is common to see one or both knees behind or in front of the line between the ankle and hip. Where the knee lies in front of the leg line, the knee has not locked out and this may often occur following injury, especially where the knee is swollen. As the knee extends for its last few degrees the knee bones twist and the tightness of the knee ligaments locks the knee (*screw home effect*). This effect stabilizes the knee and no muscle work is required to stand with the leg locked in this way. However, if the knee fails to lock completely the screw home effect will not occur, meaning that the knee has to be stabilised by continuous muscle work, a much more demanding situation. Where the knee lies behind the leg line (*genu recurvatum*) the knee has hyperextended, overstretching its posterior structures. Bear in mind that any change in the leg alignment can alter walking or running gait and have an indirect effect on either the pelvis or lumbar spine. For this reason, lower limb alignment is important to the planning of back rehabilitation.

The position of the greater trochanter, pelvis and lumbar spine is important for low back pain. Postural changes will alter the tilt of the pelvis and change the resting length of the muscles attaching to the pelvis. Over time some muscles shorten and tighten, while others lengthen and become lax. The result is *muscle imbalance.*

When the pelvis tips forwards (anterior pelvic tilt) the lumbar curve (lordosis) will *increase*

Key point:

In an optimal posture, when the knee locks straight, little or no leg muscle work is required to maintain the position.

hollowing the back. When it tips backwards (posterior pelvic tilt) the back is *flattened*. In each case there is an alteration in stress imposed on the spinal tissues, including the discs and facet joints. In an optimal posture the pelvis remains level, with a line through the anterior superior iliac spine (ASIS) at the front of the pelvis and posterior superior iliac spine (PSIS) at the back being roughly horizontal. Normal values are from 0–5 degree anterior tilt. In addition, the ASIS should be in the same vertical alignment as the pubis (*see* fig 5.2). Where alignment of these vertical and horizontal lines of the pelvis is optimal, the lumbar curve (lordosis) is shallow and even.

The shoulder should lie on the posture line in an optimal posture, but commonly it is pulled forwards due to slouching, and this body position can lead to tightness in the anterior shoulder and chest muscles. A forward lying shoulder posture can also be the result of increased curvature of the thoracic spine (thoracic kyphosis), forward tilting of the scapula, or changes in the shoulder

Key Point

In an optimal pelvic alignment, there is a *horizontal* level between the ASIS and PSIS, and a *vertical* level between the ASIS and the pubis.

joint (socket). Often several factors coexist, so close examination is vital to ensure stretching is targeted at the right structures.

The ear should rest on the posture line with the neck forming a shallow inward curve (cervical lordosis). One of the most common postural abnormalities is that of the forward head posture, where the head is thrust forwards increasing the cervical lordosis. A forward head position tightens the muscles at the base of the skull and in the upper neck, requiring a chin tuck action (*see* page 78) to stretch them.

FROM IN FRONT

Posture assessment from the front looks mainly at symmetry of muscle development and ribcage alignment. Begin looking at ankle and foot alignment to confirm your findings from postural evaluation from the side and back. Next, look at the thigh muscles (quadriceps) as asymmetry and wasting is common in those with a history of knee injury. Note also the gap between the knees to determine if your client has knock knees (genu valgum) or bow legs (genu varum). Normally the bones of the inner knee (medial condyle) and the bones of the inner ankle (medial malleolus) of each side should be close together.

The pelvis and hips should be in horizontal alignment when viewed from the front with the greater trochanters in line and the ASIS of each side also in line. Commonly one hip may drop showing as the greater trochanter lowering on that side, with the pelvis tipping away from the horizontal. Two main causes are common here: leg length discrepancy and change in hip muscle balance. Leg length changes can occur where the femur or tibia of one side are of unequal length. This may be developmental or as a result of trauma. As babies many of our bones are largely soft. As we grow the bones harden (ossify) until during adolescence we are left with bones which

Figure 5.2 Horizontal and vertical alignment of the pelvis in optimal posture

have just a small cartilage growth plate at their ends (epiphyseal plate). The growth plate is the only region of the bone, which now grows, and any injury or medical condition which damages a growth plate will stop the bone from growing any further.

> **Key point:**
>
> Changes in leg length may occur due to alteration in bone or muscle tone/length. Muscle length may be changed with stretching, bone may not.

Severe trauma such as a broken leg as a result of a road traffic accident can lead to bones healing slightly shorter than they were, so if your client has had this type of injury one leg may be shorter than the other, requiring their shoe to be built up. Clinical measures of leg length are available and the client should be referred to an orthopaedic specialist for this, as significant changes in leg length will cause a low-level but continuous stress on the spine.

Changes in leg alignment may also occur following hip pain. The side gluteal muscles (gluteus medius) hold the pelvis up when you stand on one leg. If this muscle is weak (common in the swayback posture described below) the pelvis will drop downwards when your client stands on one leg. Over time this type of asymmetry of muscle strength may lead to an alteration of posture even when standing on both legs. Your client may favour one leg and shift their pelvis over that side with little weight taken on the other side. In addition, to compensate for the horizontal tip in the pelvis the client's trunk may side bend, shortening the trunk tissues on one side and lengthening them on the other, giving the appearance of a side bent spine (scoliosis).

The ribcage should be symmetrical, but a number of changes may be seen here as well. The lower ribs should be on the same horizontal line. Where they are not, the spine may be tipped to the side or the side flexor muscles may be tighter on one side, requiring stretching (see below). Palpation is required however because some individuals have one less rib on one side compared to the other.

The sternum (breastbone) should be vertical or angled upwards slightly. Thoracic flexion (increased kyphosis) will angle the sternum down, and some individuals have an altered sternal alignment, which is developmental (funnel chest). The clavicles should be symmetrical and often changes in the scapula identified during postural assessment from behind are confirmed by looking from the front as well. Finally the head should be held straight, with tightness in the upper trapezius or sternocleidomastoid muscles typically presenting as a raised shoulder and/or side tipped head.

ASSESSING LOCAL MUSCLE TIGHTNESS

The plumb-line posture assessment described above gives us an indication of segmental alignment. From this we can predict which muscles will have poor tone (sag) and which are likely to be tight and require stretching. More precise tests will enable us to be more accurate about which individual muscles are tight, and therefore help us to be more objective with our exercise prescription.

Some of the most frequently used local clinical muscle tests are described below, and further tests are listed in Chapter 16. For all these tests, the client should be positioned ideally on an examination (massage) couch or gym bench. (For more detailed information on postural tests, *see* Norris, 1998.)

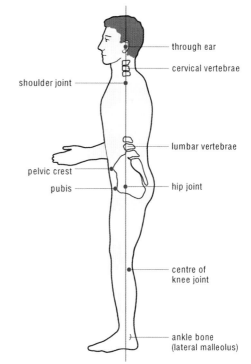

Figure 5.3 Posture plumb-line

THOMAS TEST

The Thomas test measures tightness in the hip flexors (iliopsoas and rectus femoris). The client lies on their back, with their knees bent and hanging over the end of the bench. From this position, both legs are fully flexed, bringing the knees to the chest and flattening the lumbar curve. The client holds one knee to their chest to maintain the lumbar position, and the other leg is lowered towards the horizontal, allowing the knee to extend (*see* fig 5.4). The position of the femur and tibia indicates the muscle tightness.

If the femur rests above the horizontal, the hip flexors are tighter than is desirable. Either the iliopsoas or the rectus femoris could be affected, and straightening the knee will distinguish between the two. If straightening the leg allows the femur to drop down lower, the rectus is the tighter of the two muscles. This is because the rectus works over both the knee and the hip (the iliopsoas does not work over the knee) and straightening the knee takes some of the stretch off the rectus. If the femur position remains unchanged, the iliopsoas is tighter than the rectus.

The knee, hip and shoulder should also be in line. If the femur is abducted, the ilio-tibial band (ITB) is likely to be tight. Similarly the tibia should rest vertically. If it does not, tightness in the hip rotators may be indicated.

OBER TEST

The Ober test measures tightness in the hip abductors (ilio-tibial band and gluteals) and is named after Frank Ober, who first described it in 1935. Essentially, the test aims to assess the length of the hip abductors while maintaining the neutral position of the pelvis in the frontal plane. The client lies on a bench on their side with the lower leg bent for comfort. The therapist stands behind them level with their pelvis (*see* fig 5.5). The client's leg is abducted and extended to 15 degrees and the pelvis is stabilised to prevent lateral tilting. The therapist presses down on the client's pelvic rim, with their left hand angling the push towards the client's lower shoulder. The therapist's right hand supports the weight of the abducted upper leg. While preventing any pelvic movement, the upper leg is lowered down, keeping it slightly back. Normally, the leg should lower to the horizontal position before any pelvic movement is detected. In an athlete, the leg should lower to the couch top, indicating that

> **Key point:**
>
> The Ober test measures tightness in the ilio-tibial (ITB) of the upper lying leg.

Figure 5.4 Thomas test: (a) knee is gripped to the chest and the opposite leg should touch the couch and show 90° flexion; (b) tight hip flexors; (c) tight abductors (ITB)

Figure 5.5 Ober test

the ITB and gluteals possess adequate flexibility. If the leg stops above the horizontal position, or if pelvic movement begins with the leg in this upper position, the ITB is tight. This test is also described in chapter 10, exercise 92, page 155.

TRIPOD TEST

There are many tests to assess the length of the hamstrings, including the straight leg raise and active knee extension exercises. The tripod test, however, measures both hamstring tightness and the effect of any tightness on pelvic tilt and low back alignment.

Figure 5.6 Tripod test: (a) pelvis level, leg straightens; (b) tight hamstrings cause backwards pelvic tilt and lumbar flexion

The client sits on the edge of a bench with the feet unsupported. The spine is placed in its neutral position (*see* page 75) with the lower back slightly hollow. From this position, one leg is straightened and the alignment of the lumbo-pelvic area is noted (*see* fig 5.6). Ideally, the leg should be straightened to 70–80 degrees while maintaining spinal alignment. Often, the leg cannot be fully straightened, and the spine sags into flexion, posteriorly tilting the pelvis and flexing the lumbar region. This is important because it indicates that tightness in the hamstrings is dictating spinal alignment, which is a common cause of postural back pain. As well as hamstring stretching exercises, core stability exercises should be practised to correct the fault.

ANTERIOR CHEST TEST

Tightness in the pectorals and anterior deltoids will cause the shoulders to be pulled forwards, and is assessed with the client lying on their back. Their arm is taken out to the side into a 'T' position (*see* fig 5.7(a)) and ideally should rest level with the bench. Taking the arm diagonally so that it lies on the horizontal (frontal plane) and at 45 degrees to the spine, will stress the sternal fibres of the pectoralis major and anterior deltoid (*see* fig 5.7(b)). Taking the arm back to the 'T' position and then lowering the arm down the side of the bench will stress the clavicular fibres of the pectoralis major (*see* fig 5.7(c)). In this position, the arm should lie at 70–80 degrees to the chest.

The shoulder can also be pulled forwards by tightness in the pectoralis minor, which attaches from the upper ribs to the corocoid process of the scapula. When this is the case, the back of the shoulder is pulled off the bench in supine lying. Normally, the back of the shoulder should be no more than two to three finger breadths from the bench.

Figure 5.7 Anterior chest test: (a) 'T' position; (b) stressing the sternal fibres of pectoralis major and the anterior deltoid; (c) stressing the clavicular fibres of pectoralis major

SHOULDER ADDUCTORS

Tightness in the shoulder adductors (latissimus dorsi and pectoralis major) will limit arm abduction. The latissimus is measured in a supine lying position. The arm is laterally rotated (because the muscle is a medial rotator) and abducted in an attempt to take it behind the ear. Normally, the arm should rest flat on the floor (*see* fig 5.8). Refer to the 'Anterior chest test' for assessment of the pectoralis major.

POSTURAL FAULTS AND CORRECTION

ENHANCING CORE STABILITY

Before we begin to correct postural faults with stretching, we must ensure that an individual can hold firmly the origin of the muscles to be stretched. If this is not done, when we stretch both ends of the muscle will move and alignment will be poor. Many of the large muscles of the lower limbs attach to the lumbo-pelvic region, while many muscles of the upper limbs attach to the scapula. Both of these areas must be stabilised before stretching begins.

The neutral spine position

The lumbo-pelvic region is stabilised by the deep abdominal muscles (transversus abdominis and internal oblique). Looking at figure 5.9, we can see that the superficial abdominals (rectus abdominis and external oblique) have fibres which run more or less vertically while the deep abdominals have largely horizontal fibres. When the muscles pull, therefore, the superficial abdominals will pull the pelvis to the ribcage (flexion or rotation), while the deep abdominals will pull the abdominal wall to the spine and 'tighten the girdle'. In this way the deep abdominals are more able to stabilise the trunk and hold it in a 'neutral position' – mid-way between flexion (flat back) and extension (hollow back) (*see* fig 5.10). The neutral position aligns the lumbar tissues optimally and places least stress upon them.

When we move away from the neutral position, stress is increased. As we increase the hollow of the lumbar spine, the facet joints at the back of the spine are compressed. Over time, this can cause pain and joint damage, possibly leading to wear and tear of the joints themselves. If we reduce the hollow in the back, the spine is flexed and stress moves from the facet joints on to the disc.

Key point:

The neutral position of the lumber spine lies mid-way between forward (hollow back) and backward (flat back) tilting of the pelvis.

Figure 5.8 Measuring tightness in the latissimus dorsi: full abduction is combined with lateral rotation

The flexion stress compresses the disc, tending to force it on to the nerves of the lower spine. This type of posture can give pain through nerve compression or nerve entrapment.

HOW TO FIND YOUR NEUTRAL SPINE POSITION

To find the neutral position of the lower spine, we begin standing upright. Tilt the pelvis backwards, forcing your spine to flex (flatten) and then tilt your pelvis forwards, extending (hollowing) your spine. The neutral position is mid-way between fully flattening and fully hollowing the spine. It should be the most comfortable position, depending on your posture type. (Posture types are discussed in detail later in this chapter.)

CORE STABILITY EXERCISES

Having found the neutral position, we perform a series of simple exercises to re-educate the core stability muscles. First, we have to regain the hollowing function of the abdominals. Many people find this difficult initially, and tend to bend the spine instead.

Abdominal hollowing in standing

Start by standing up straight (*see* fig 5.11). Focus your attention on your tummy button (umbilicus) and tighten your abdominal muscles to pull your

Figure 5.9 The abdominal muscles

tummy button in. A number of faults can occur when performing this exercise (*see* fig 5.12). First, be careful not to take a deep breath or hold your breath, and do not flex the spine. If you look at your lower ribs, they should not move throughout the hollowing action. If the ribs are drawn down, the superficial abdominals are working instead of the deep abdominals. If the ribs lift up, you are simply taking a deep breath and pulling your abdominal wall tight using respiration rather than abdominal muscle action.

Abdominal hollowing in kneeling

Allow your abdominal wall to sag down, and then pull it tight and up as if trying to touch your tummy button to your spine. Again, make sure it is only your abdominal wall that is moving. Do not move your spine or hips (*see* fig 5.13).

Heel slide

When you have mastered the abdominal hollowing exercises, you are ready to hold your spine stable

Figure 5.10 Neutral position of the lumbar spine: (a) neutral positions; (b) hollow back – facet joints compact; (c) flat back – disc is stressed

Figure 5.11 Abdominal hollowing in standing

Figure 5.12 Common faults in abdominal hollowing in standing: (a) the distance from the lower ribs to the pelvis (X) remains unchanged; (b) taking a deep breath: the ribs move up increasing (X); (c) flexing the trunk, the ribs move down, decreasing (X)

Figure 5.13 (a) and (b) Abdominal hollowing in kneeling

Figure 5.14 Heel slide

against resistance. In the heel slide (*see* fig 5.14), the hip flexor muscles are pulling on your spine, trying to move it away from the neutral position, while you are using your deep abdominal muscles to try to prevent the movement and maintain stability.

Lie on your back with your knees bent and place your arms by your sides. Pull your lower abdominals tight (hollowing) as before and keep them tight throughout the movement, without holding your breath. Slide one of your legs out straight, making sure that your pelvis does not move and your spine does not hollow. You should aim to perform 10 slow repetitions on each leg, with each complete single leg movement taking about 10 seconds. No pelvic movement at all should occur throughout the whole exercise sequence.

To make it easier to spot unwanted pelvic movement, work with a partner. Place an adhesive marker on the front part of the upper lip of your pelvis (the anterior superior iliac spine) or mark it with a felt-tip pen. This will make it easier for your partner to detect even the smallest amount of pelvic movement.

HOLLOW-BACK POSTURE

The lower part of the back (the lumbar spine) should normally be slightly hollow. This curve (the lumbar lordosis) is greatly affected by the tilt of the pelvis. The pelvis is balanced like a see-saw on the hip joints, and is controlled by the abdominal, spinal and hip muscles, and the ligaments that surround these areas. The abdominal muscles, working together with the gluteals and hamstrings, will tilt the pelvis backwards and flatten the lower spine, while the hip flexors and spinal extensors will tilt the pelvis forwards and increase the lumbar curve.

Pelvic crossed syndrome

In many cases an imbalance of these muscles exists, known as the *pelvic crossed syndrome* (PCS). Here we see a combination of excessive length and weakness in the abdominal muscles and gluteals (sagging) and tightness in the spinal extensors and iliopsoas (*see* fig 5.15). The pelvis is seen to tip forwards, pulling the lumbar spine into

Figure 5.15 Pelvic crossed syndrome (PCS)

Key point:

In the hollow back posture, the abdominal muscles and gluteals are lax (saggy), while the hip flexors and low back are tight.

an increased curvature or lordosis. This, in turn, causes stress to the small facet joints deep within the lumbar spine. This is the classic 'beer belly' posture, also seen after pregnancy and as a result of abdominal surgery.

The weakness of the gluteal muscles has an important bearing on walking and running. Normally, as we take a step and the hip moves into extension, the gluteal muscles contract powerfully to push the body forwards. However, in PCS these muscles are weak and so are unable to propel the body correctly. To compensate for this, the hamstring muscles contract in an attempt to do the work of the gluteals (the hamstrings eventually becoming tight themselves). Because the hamstrings are not as strong as the gluteals, the action of hip extension is weaker. The body tries to make up for this by extending the lumbar spine instead of the hip, and again stress is placed on the lumbar region. The appearance now when running, stepping and walking is of a 'duck waddle' around the pelvic region.

How to correct the pelvic crossed syndrome

To correct this syndrome, we cannot simply strengthen the gluteal muscles, because the imbalance affects all of the hip muscles. Instead, we must first focus our attention on stretching the tight hip flexor muscles. We saw on page 38 that there is a relationship between antagonistic pairs of muscles: when one muscle contracts, its opposite must relax. In the case of the hip muscles, the tight hip flexors have greater muscle tone and, therefore, may actually reduce the potential tone and strength of the hip extensors that lie opposite. This action of reducing tone by 'inhibition' (fewer nerve impulses reaching the muscle) is also known as *pseudoparesis* and is an important factor in balancing muscle pull around a joint. In the case of PCS, we must stretch the iliopsoas and hamstrings (*see* table 5.2,(a) and (b)) while maintaining a neutral spine position. Once this has been achieved, both the gluteals and the lower abdominal muscles must be re-strengthened to correct the pelvic tilt. It is

Table 5.2	Stretching exercises for posture
Problem	**Exercise**
(a) Tight hip flexors	Iliopsoas: hold on to an object for stability and press your hips forwards
(b) Tight hamstrings	Hamstrings: hold the back of one leg and straighten it
(c) Head appears to be held forwards, poking chin	Chin tuck: place hand on chin and gently slide head back horizontally
(d) Tight band from neck to shoulder (upper trapezius), head appears tilted to one side	Side bend: fix the shoulders by gripping a chair and pull the head in the opposite direction
(e) Round shoulders	'Pec stretch': stand in the corner of a room, place the arms on a wall and lean forwards
(f) Flat low back	Low back: push up on to the elbows
(g) Tight back when bending forwards	Low back: grip the knees into the chest

important to work the abdominals in their inner range to shorten, rather than simply strengthen, the muscles. Details of abdominal work of this type may be found in *The Complete Guide to Abdominal Training* (Christopher M. Norris, A & C Black, London, 2009).

KYPHOTIC POSTURE
Upper crossed syndrome

An imbalance pattern also exists around the shoulder girdle, known as the *upper crossed syndrome* (UCS). Here the upper trapezius, levator scapulae and pectoral muscles are tight, while the deep neck flexors and the lower scapular stabilisers (serratus anterior and lower trapezius) are inhibited and weak. The abnormal posture seen here is one in which the head is held forwards (poking chin) and the normal curve in the neck is flattened out. This head posture places stress on the neck tissues and frequent headaches can result. The shoulders are rounded and the scapulae move further apart. In some cases, the scapulae can be seen standing prominent under the skin (winging). Tightness in the trapezius and levator scapulae is commonly seen as a straightening of the neck/shoulder line, where the muscles stand out like tight cords (*see* fig 5.16). This posture is frequently seen in those who spend many hours slumped over a desk and do little exercise in their spare time.

The altered muscular control of the scapulae causes them to twist slightly so that the shoulder socket (glenoid fossa) faces more vertically than normal. This means that the shoulder muscles must work harder to stop the joint from dislocating, and this additional work can give rise to a painful 'frozen shoulder' over time.

Although the shoulder girdle is a separate structure from the thoracic spine, the shoulder posture in UCS pulls the thoracic spine into excessive flexion, forcing the ribs together anteriorly and making breathing more difficult. In some cases, the thoracic vertebrae soften and develop incorrectly, a condition called

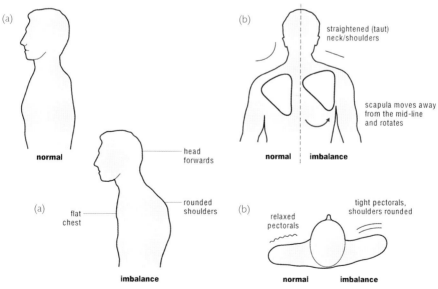

Figure 5.16 Upper crossed syndrome (UCS)

Scheuermann's disease, which requires specialist treatment. In this case, the shoulder posture results from the spinal posture rather than the other way round.

Figure 5.17 Shoulder stability exercises: (a) static reposition; (b) sternal lift

---

Key point:

In the kyphotic (round shouldered) posture, the chest muscles are tight and short and the shoulder bracing muscles are lax.

How to correct upper crossed syndrome

Just as with the lower limbs, we begin the exercises by improving core stability. This time it is the stability of the shoulder blade (scapula) we are concerned with. It tends to ride up and outwards, and we need to pull it in the opposite direction. The first exercise (*see* fig 5.17(a)) is to sit on a stool and ask your training partner to pull your shoulder into its optimal alignment. The shoulder blade is pulled down and in until its inner edge is vertical and the two blades are about 12–18 cm apart. You 'set' your shoulder muscles to hold this position as your training partner releases the shoulder blade. Try to hold the position for 10–30 seconds. For the next exercise (*see* fig 5.17(b)), you try to correct your own posture and hold it. Again begin sitting, but try to lift your breastbone (sternum) without taking a deep breath. At the same time draw your shoulder blade in and down. Hold the position for 10–30 seconds as before, breathing normally.

When the kyphotic posture is created by tissue tightness alone, stretching is called for. Stretching is aimed at the neck (*see* table 5.2 (c)), the levator scapulae and upper trapezius (*see* table 5.2 (d)) and the pectoral and anterior deltoid muscles (*see* table 5.2 (e)). In each case, the scapula is stabilised in its optimal position (down and in) throughout the stretch.

In many cases, the lordotic (hollow back) posture and the kyphotic posture may occur together (kypho-lordosis). This is because the increase in the lumbar lordosis results in an increased kyphosis to compensate, which brings the bodyweight back over the plumb-line. If this is the case, exercise therapy must be aimed at both areas.

SWAY-BACK POSTURE

In a sway-back posture, the whole pelvis moves forwards and the hips are forced into extension. While the pelvic tilt remains, the thoracic spine flexes and the lumbar lordosis is increased. This stresses the hip ligaments and the ligaments on the front of the lower spine and behind the thoracic spine.

Comparing normal and sway-back postures (*see* fig 5.18), we can see that in the case of normal posture the furthest point forwards is the chest, and the furthest backwards is the buttocks. In the case of sway-back posture, the furthest point forwards

Figure 5.18 Sway-back posture

Key point:

The sway-back is the 'slouch' posture. The pelvis drifts forwards and the body height is reduced. The key to correction is to 'stand tall'.

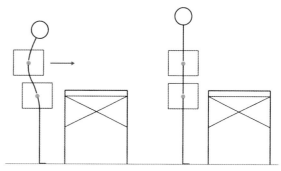

Figure 5.19 Correcting the sway-back posture

is the abdomen and the furthest backwards is the thoracic spine. In the normal posture, the lumbar curve is gently hollow along the whole length of the lumbar spine. In the sway-back posture, the hollow is sharp and more pronounced in the lower area. Finally, in the normal posture the spine and legs are close to the plumb-line, but in the sway-back posture the spine and legs form a curve.

The sway-back tends to be a temporary 'slouching' posture, frequently seen in adolescents as they suddenly start to grow tall and 'shoot up'. However, it is still a cause of pain when held for longer periods. Correction involves tucking the chin in and lengthening the spine as though you were a puppet on a rope hanging from the ceiling. In addition, the chest should move forwards while the pelvis remains still. The easiest way to learn is by standing in front of a table and imagining

the pelvis and chest as two toy building blocks sliding on top of each other (*see* fig 5.19). The hips should not touch the table, and the chest should slide forwards as one unit, without altering spinal alignment.

FLAT-BACK POSTURE

The flat-back posture shows a markedly reduced lumbar lordosis, and is commonly seen with those who sit for prolonged periods in their job. It is also common following back pain when a person has rested in bed. The individual is unable to move the spine correctly, and most of the structures around it are stiff and sore. Stiffness may limit either flexion or extension, and the spine becomes almost fixed in a flat-back position. Stretching can help to alleviate the pain from this condition as the lost flexibility is gradually regained. The stretches should feel slightly uncomfortable, because they are working on very tight structures; however, they should not give back pain. If they do, exercise should be carried out only under the supervision of a physiotherapist.

With the flat-back posture the spine is gradually stretched into extension (*see* table 5.2 (f)). When forward bending is also limited, flexion stretches may be performed using the hips for leverage (*see* table 5.2 (g)). In each case, the movement is gently encouraged rather than being vigorously forced.

Key point:

The flat-back is the classic sitting posture. With prolonged sitting, a person almost becomes 'chair-shaped'. The lumbar curve is lost and the hips are tight and immobile.

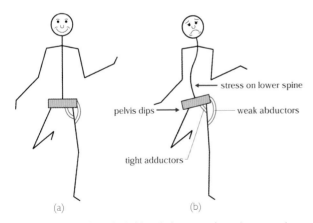

(a) (b)

Figure 5.20 Weak hip abductors alter the stepping gait: (a) normal muscle balance – abductors and adductors are the same length and strength; (b) imbalance – tight hip adductors inhibit (weaken) abductors. As the opposite foot is lifted from the ground, weak abductors fail to support the pelvis, allowing it to dip down.

POSTURAL FAULTS IN THE LOWER LIMBS

Postural faults in the foot and leg can be detrimental to knee health, and stretching can help to alleviate the faults. We have seen that imbalance between the various hip and lumbar spine muscles can alter the way in which the hip is extended when walking and running. A further imbalance pattern also exists between the hip abductor and adductor muscles. The adductors show a tendency to tighten, and this in turn inhibits the hip abductors. The abductor muscles are important stabilisers of the pelvis as we lift one leg from the ground, as in walking, stepping and running. As we lift the leg, the abductor muscles (especially gluteus medius) of the leg on the ground work hard to prevent the pelvis from dipping down. If these muscles are inhibited and weak, the pelvis dips, causing a sideways 'duck waddle' (*see* fig 5.20). This is most noticeable when performing step aerobics.

We saw in the PCS that when the hip extensors are weak, the hamstring muscles work by substitution, and in so doing they become tight. In the case of weak hip abductors, the tensor fascia lata muscle works instead. This muscle attaches to the ilio-tibial band (ITB), which travels down the side of the leg. The ITB, in turn, has a connection to the side of the knee with a small slip to the kneecap itself. Because the tensor fascia lata is having to work too hard to cover up for the weakened hip abductors, it tightens the ITB and pulls the kneecap outwards as weight is taken on one leg. This is a very common cause of a painful kneecap, often seen in sport.

Correcting lower limb postural faults

The action now is clear. First, we must stretch the tight hip adductors. Then, if the condition has been present for some time, the ITB will be tight and will need to be stretched using the Ober

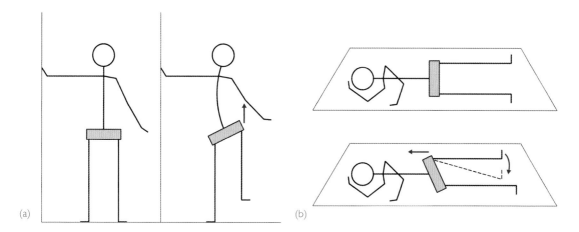

Figure 5.21 Self-stretch of tight hip abductors: (a) hip hitching in standing; (b) abductor stretch after hip hitching

Key point:

When we stand on one leg, the adductor muscles of the weight-bearing leg 'hitch' the pelvis up, preventing it from sagging.

side flexors are tightened by the hip hitching action. These muscles should remain tight as the upper leg is lowered, to prevent any lateral tilting of the pelvis. The stretch is felt over the outside of the hip.

test (*see* page 72). The test is performed, and the position of maximum stretch with the leg near the horizontal is held for 10–20 seconds. This should be practised daily with 5–8 repetitions.

To perform this technique without a partner requires good lateral stability of the pelvis. This may be assessed using a 'hip hitching', or 'leg shortening', exercise (*see* fig 5.21). With hip hitching in standing (*see* fig 5.21(a)) the athlete stands side-on to a wall with the near hand on the wall to aid balance. Keeping both legs straight, the action is to shorten one leg so that the pelvis moves upwards on the short leg side. In the side lying position, the upper leg is again abducted and slightly extended. From this position, the trunk

SUMMARY

- In a good posture, the body segments are aligned to minimise joint stress.
- A good posture requires minimal muscle work to maintain.
- Posture is assessed with reference to a 'plumb-line' from behind and the side.
- Local tests of muscle tightness are used to determine postural problems in specific parts of the body.
- Posture correction begins by enhancing a person's core stability.
- A muscle imbalance correction programme is used to stretch tight muscle and strengthen/shorten lax muscle in order to realign the body segments.

STRETCHING RESEARCH

6

In this chapter we will look at some of the research that has been conducted on the aspects of stretching covered in the rest of the book. Research is ongoing, so knowledge in this subject area is always increasing. Full details of recent research papers are listed in the reference section on pages 281–283.

STRETCHING AND POSTURE

In a lordotic posture, the pelvis is anteriorly tilted and 'hangs on the hamstrings'. In this posture, the hamstrings are likely to be tight (increased tone), whereas in other postures their length is likely to be unrelated to pelvic tilt. Li et al., (1996) measured the importance of the length of the hamstrings. They took subjects with tight hamstrings who had a straight leg raise (SLR) of less than 70 degrees, and then applied a stretching programme. They found that the SLR improved and the motion of the pelvis in forward bending changed. Interestingly, the static postural alignment of the pelvis did not alter.

The importance of the pelvic tilt position when performing a hamstring stretch was addressed by Sullivan et al., (1992). They took 20 subjects with tight hamstrings and used static stretching and PNF techniques in either anterior or posterior pelvic tilt. Each subject performed 10 minutes of

stretching for four days per week over a two-week period. They found that the group who used a starting position of anterior pelvic tilt gained significantly greater hamstring flexibility.

> **Key point:**
>
> The length of the hamstrings is more important to pelvic control during forward bending than to static posture itself. When stretching the hamstrings, performing the exercise with an anterior pelvic tilt gives better results.

STRETCHING AND MUSCLE STIFFNESS

Halbertsma et al., (1996) looked at the load–deformation curve (see page 15) of stretched muscle. They took subjects with slightly short hamstrings (SLR less than 80 degrees) and applied 10 minutes of static stretching for a single period. They found that the stress strain curves before and after exercise did not change, indicating that the stiffness of the muscle did not change in a single exercise bout; however, the range of motion increased.

To measure the effect of stretching on muscle stiffness, McNair and Stanley (1996) used oscillation of the calf muscles. In their experimental set-up, subjects were seated with a weight on their knee and their foot on a rocker mechanism that allowed their heel to drop down into dorsiflexion, pre-stretching their calf muscles. Another weight was then dropped on the knee to rapidly stretch their muscles further. An accelerometer was connected to the weight holder resting on the leg to measure vertical movement and oscillation. The small movements that occurred were amplified 100 times, and an EMG recording demonstrated that no voluntary muscle contraction was occurring.

They found, first, that the elastic stiffness of the calf muscles reduced significantly after 10 minutes' jogging at 60 per cent of maximal heart rate; and that, second, the same effect was achieved after static stretching for 5 repetitions, holding each stretch for 30 seconds with a 30-second rest between each stretch.

Measuring the effect of tendon tap on the calf muscles was used to demonstrate the effect of stretching on muscle reflexes by Rosenbaum and Henning (1995). They showed improved muscle compliance after 3 minutes of static stretching of the calf muscles, and improved muscle force development and decreased EMG activity after a 10-minute warm-up run on a treadmill.

Magnusson et al., (1996) used the movement of an isokinetic dynamometer (passive torque) to measure the resistance of the hamstring muscles to stretch during passive knee extension. Passive torque is the force that a muscle exerts to 'push back' against the pressure of the machine. The subjects in the study performed a static hamstrings stretch, holding the stretch for 90 seconds. They performed 5 repetitions of this movement with a 30-second rest between each stretch. During the static stretch, passive torque reduced, indicating

that the muscles were 'giving' a little. The stiffness of the muscles was also shown to reduce, but both measures returned to normal within one hour of testing.

> **Key point:**
>
> Static stretching has been shown to improve stretch tolerance, reduce muscle stiffness, and produce muscle changes, which would tend to reduce the risk of injury.

STRETCHING AS PART OF A WARM-UP

A warm-up will result in a number of physiological factors that may be of benefit to stretching. Elevated temperature improves a person's ability to perform physical work in general as the critical level at which various metabolic chemical reactions occur is lower, so the reactions occur sooner (Bergh and Ekblom, 1979). In addition, muscle contraction is more rapid and more forceful (Bergh, 1980). The sensitivity of nerve receptors and the speed at which a nerve is able to transmit its impulse is quicker (Astrand and Rodahl, 1986). The improvements in nerve conduction seen after a warm-up are particularly important for PNF stretching, for example, where reflex mechanisms are used to improve range of motion.

The stiffness (viscosity) of the synovial fluid limits a joint's range and ease of motion. The viscosity of the synovial fluid is reduced meaning that it offers less resistance, as its temperature rises during a warm-up (Astrand and Rodahl, 1986). A greater force and length of stretch is required to tear muscle that has undergone a warm-up, due to the reduction in viscosity of the connective tissue within the muscle (Safran et al., 1988).

LaBan (1962) showed a 1.5 per cent increase in the length of a stretched tendon following a temperature increase to 42.5°C, while Warren et al., (1971) demonstrated that a tendon heated to 45°C increased in length by 5.8 per cent and its force to failure was 58 per cent greater than that at a normal body temperature. Realistically, these extreme temperatures, compared to a normal body temperature of 38.9°C, can only be achieved through passive heating as used by a physiotherapist. However, they do demonstrate the importance of allowing tissue to warm before it is stretched.

EFFECTS OF TEMPERATURE ON PLIABILITY OF BODY TISSUE

When a tissue is warmed, it takes a greater stretching force to tear it (Safran et al., 1988) due to a change in the resistance offered by the tissue, known as its 'viscoelastic' property. In the sixties and seventies, early research work demonstrated this effect quite clearly. Tendons could be stretched further before rupturing (LaBan, 1962) and a 50–60 per cent greater force was needed before the tendon actually failed and tore (Warren et al., 1971).

Ice also affects tissue pliability. When applied to the skin, ice causes a reduction in blood flow to the superficial tissues, but also causes a reddening of the skin (hyperaemia) as a protective effect. Following injury, the reduction of blood flow is used to slow the metabolic rate of the injured tissues and limit any damage caused by the injury. In terms of stretching, however, the important feature of ice application is that it depresses muscle spindle activity, an important component of the stretch reflex (Halvorson, 1990). Muscle spasm is reduced, and the muscle itself takes on a more relaxed state.

It must be remembered that the effect of ice is more likely to be reflex in nature, as the cold does not go very deeply into the body tissues. On the skin, the temperature reduction may be as much as 20°C after ice application for 20 minutes (Palmer and Knight 1996), but at a depth of only 1.7 cm the change in temperature reduces dramatically to 4°C (Zemke et al., 1998). In a joint, temperature reduction is unlikely, except for the superficial joints of the toes and fingers. Levy and Lintner (1997) found no significant temperature reduction in the shoulder (glenohumeral) joint, even after 90 minutes of ice application.

Key point:

When used as part of a warm-up, stretching has beneficial effects on muscle, tendon, nerve and joint structures.

DOES HEAT OR ICE IMPROVE STRETCHING TECHNIQUES?

Heat applied before static stretching does not result in a greater increase in range of motion from a hamstring stretch (Taylor et al., 1995). When applied together with a static stretch, however, the story can be different, resulting in an increased range of motion at the hip, shoulder and shin (Shrier and Gossal, 2000). Ice applied in combination with a static stretch (cryostretch) is most effective when applied in the early stages of stretching (Lentell et al., 1992). However, the effect of cryostretch seems more appropriate to muscles in spasm through pain or injury.

On normal muscle, heat and cold do not seem to improve the effectiveness of stretching. Using an active knee extension (AKE) stretch, Taylor et al., (1995) examined static stretching alone and static stretching with either heat or cold;

they found no difference between any of the groups. Cornelius et al., (1992) came to a similar conclusion concerning PNF stretching; they looked at static stretching and PNF stretching, with and without cold application, and found no significant differences between the groups.

INJURY PREVENTION

Many athletes believe that a warm-up and stretching will help to prevent injury and make them perform better. If stretching can offer less resistance to movement and increase range of motion, it is possible to see that a mechanism may exist to justify these claims. However, because there are many factors interrelated with injury and performance, these claims are as yet to be fully substantiated.

The combination of warm-up and stretching has been shown by some authors to actually reduce the incidence of injury. Ekstrand et al., (1983) showed that a group of footballers performing a

20-minute warm-up, which included 10 minutes of stretching, suffered only 75 per cent of the injuries that their colleagues, who did not perform the warm-up, did. Stretching as part of a rehabilitation programme has also been shown to reduce the rate of injury recurrence to only 1 per cent following calf muscle injury (Millar, 1976).

Stretching may also improve the efficiency of movement in certain circumstances. In one study (Godges et al., 1989), the economy of running gait was shown to improve at both moderate and high exercise intensities through increases in hip range of motion thanks to stretching exercises. Other studies, however, have shown the reverse. Gleim et al., (1990) showed that 'tighter' subjects were significantly more economical as fast walkers and joggers than more flexible subjects. The tighter subjects also demonstrated better oxygen consumption values on treadmill activities.

Research by Krivickas and Feinberg (1996) tested 200 college athletes and found that the risk of injury decreased as flexibility improved. These authors showed a 15 per cent increased risk of injury for those who were less flexible and a 20 per cent reduced risk for those who were more flexible. However, the opposite was found by Askling et al., (2002) when looking at hamstring flexibility in ballet dancers; they showed that stretching could give rise to injury in the upper portion of the hamstrings. In a study of over 1500 army recruits over a 12-week period, Pope et al., (2000) found 158 injuries in those who stretched and 175 in those who did not, but, when analysed statistically, the results showed no significant difference between the stretching and non-stretching (control) group.

Some authors have investigated the stretching studies themselves to determine the quality of the research involved. A study by two Australian physiotherapists (Herbert and Gabriel, 2002) summarised the information gained from five scientific studies, and concluded that there was no evidence that stretching – either before or after exercise – protects against muscle soreness or injury. In a later study, two UK-based osteopaths (Weldon and Hill, 2003) conducted a review of seven papers and decided that no definitive conclusions could be made concerning the value of stretching due to the poor quality of the available studies. However, a systematic review by Fradkin et al., (2006) looked at papers (all high-quality randomised controlled trials) between 1966 and 2005, and concluded that 'the weight of evidence is in favour of decreased risk of injury'.

The jury is certainly still out on this one. Athletes and coaches often believe that stretching is beneficial in some way as regards injury prevention, but the research is yet to determine first, if any benefit exists, and second, how any such benefit could be obtained. Based on the current research, the recommendation must be that, before physical exertion of any type, an active warm-up to increase both tissue and joint temperature is probably better than simply static stretching alone. In addition, a specific warm-up to match the movement patterns of the sport to be undertaken is likely to optimally prepare the athlete from the point of view of motor control (Shrier, 2000, Shrier and Gossal, 2000).

If stretching does prevent injury, how is this achieved? This was a problem addressed by a team from Ghent University in Belgium (Witvrouw et al., 2004) who considered the type of activity to be one of the most important factors in determining whether stretching was effective at preventing injuries or not. Exercises which require bouncing and jumping activities (plyometrics, *see* page 37) require the muscle-tendon unit to be springy and compliant, in other words less 'stiff'. This, as we have seen, is a feature which stretching can achieve. If athletes performing these tasks have a stiffer muscle-tendon unit, the demands placed on it by high-intensity exercise may exceed the tissue capacity, causing injury. In those athletes who use only low-intensity exercise (jogging for example) there may be no advantage to having a muscle-tendon unit which is less stiff, and so injury prevention is not likely to be seen here.

Key point:

Long-term stretching reduces stiffness in the muscle-tendon unit which may be protective in some power sports.

MUSCLE REFLEXES AND STRETCHING

The effects of stretching on muscle reflexes are often investigated by measuring the excitability of a muscle. To do this, a Hoffmann reflex (H reflex) is used. We saw that, when a muscle is stretched rapidly, it responds by evoking a stretch reflex (*see* page 56). The Hoffman reflex is similar, except that it is an artificial reflex. If a muscle, usually the soleus in the calf, is electrically stimulated with a single shock, a muscle twitch results and is seen on an EMG machine. The strength of this muscle twitch (H reflex) is recorded as the height of the EMG signal graph. If a group of motor nerve cells (motor neuron pool) is more active (excitable),

Key point:

Before sport, use an active warm-up to increase both tissue and joint temperature, and a specific warm-up to match the movement patterns of the sport.

the H reflex will be stronger because more motor nerves are involved in the contraction.

A number of factors will influence the excitability of the motor neuron pool. For example, if a subject clenches their teeth by biting hard, the H reflex is stronger, demonstrating that the motor nerves to all muscle will be excited. Although there is no logical connection from the jaw to the calf, there is a functional relationship that is important to stretching. When we grip any muscle tightly, in this case the jaw, neural signals are sent not just to the muscle concerned, but along the spinal cord as well. This has the effect of 'setting' the muscles and bracing our posture to create stability. This effect, known as the Jendrassik manoeuvre, is important, because if we are trying to stretch a muscle using PNF techniques, we want that muscle to relax and offer less resistance to the stretching force. If we place a subject in a starting position where they are unbalanced and gripping on to something, or where they feel insecure, the increased tone that results will have a knock-on effect to the tone of the muscle we are stretching, even though that muscle may be some distance away.

Research into the response of muscle to PNF stretching has used the H reflex to assess muscle excitability after isometric contraction using the contract–relax method (*see* page 61). Moore and Kukulka (1991) showed the H reflex to be suppressed after isometric contraction. The excitability of the motor nerve and of the stretch reflex mechanism itself appears to decrease following isometric contractions, and this decreased level lasts for about 10 seconds, whether or not the muscle was contracted for one second or 30 seconds. This gives a 10-second 'window' in which to apply the stretch.

Looking at the EMG trace to judge the efficiency of the stretch reflex, Nicol et al., (1996) used a maximum vertical depth jump. They found that both reflex activity and muscle biochemistry changed considerably: creatine kinase activity increased, showing micro-damage to the muscle fibres (as occurs with eccentric exercise); the stretch reflex sensitivity was reduced completely by the second day after exhaustive exercise; and recovery was not fully complete until four days after the exercise.

Key point:

Exhaustive exercise, especially that which is likely to cause muscle damage, such as eccentric actions, reduces the sensitivity of the stretch reflex and may remove some of its protective function. This makes injury more likely.

TYPES OF STRETCHING

Several researchers have asked the question, 'Which is the best way to stretch?' Static stretching seems to be as effective as ballistic stretching, except that ballistic stretching creates a considerable amount of muscle soreness (Etnyre and Abraham, 1986). PNF techniques provide greater improvements in range of motion than either static or ballistic methods (Enoka, 1994).

Webright et al., (1997) compared static stretching with active stretching. They took 40 subjects through a stretching programme in a sitting position. Initially, subjects were unable to lock their knee (minimum of 15 degrees short of full extension) when sitting with the femur at 90 degrees and statically stretching the hamstrings. One group practised static stretching (a single repetition held for 30 seconds), while the other practised slow (non-ballistic) active knee extension (30 repetitions, each taking one second).

Each group performed two bouts of stretching daily for six weeks. The results showed that both groups developed an equal amount of flexibility, with the subjects changing from 15 degrees short of full extension to 8–10 degrees short of full extension. Importantly, this programme demonstrated significant increases in flexibility in just six weeks through a short (30-second) stretching programme performed daily.

Key point:

PNF stretching gives superior gains in range of motion, and even brief stretching programmes (of any type) are effective, providing they are practised regularly.

STRETCHES – HOW LONG AND HOW MANY?

The exact amount of time needed to effectively stretch has been the subject of many studies. Bandy and Irion (1994) used knee extension to test static stretch timing. They chose 47 subjects with limited knee extension and subjected them to 15-, 30-, or 60-second static stretches. Each group stretched for five days a week over a period of six weeks. Their results showed that both the 30- and 60-second stretches were more effective than the 15-second stretch, but, importantly, the 60-second stretch gave no greater gains than the 30-second one. The conclusion they made was that there is no advantage in holding a stretch for 60 seconds; 30 seconds seems to be an adequate period to hold a static stretch.

Because the effects of stretching are cumulative (*see* page 52), a number of repetitions are normally performed. Taylor et al., (1990) found that the greatest effects of stretch to the muscle and

Key point:

Optimal stretching timing is 4–5 repetitions, holding each repetition for 30 seconds.

tendon occurred during the first four stretches, with a greater number of repetitions failing to produce greater improvements. In this case, more did not seem to be better!

LIMITING FACTORS IN RANGE OF MOVEMENT

Two factors limit the possible range of motion available at a joint: contractile and non-contractile structures. The degree of limitation presented by the various tissues varies between joints. In the spine, Adams et al., (1980) looked at cadavers and found that the vertebral disc limits flexion and extension movements by 29 per cent, while the supraspinous and interspinous ligaments limit the same movement by 19 per cent. The facet joint capsules have the greatest limitation to movement, at 39 per cent. For the metacarpophalangeal joints, the capsule limits movement by 47 per cent, muscle by 41 per cent, tendons by 10 per cent and skin by 2 per cent (Johns and Wright, 1992).

When muscles are relaxed, the improvement in range of motion with each successive stretch will increase. Taylor et al., (1990) used the extensor digitorum longus muscle in the leg, stretched it by a set amount and held the stretch for 30 seconds. Each bout of stretches consisted of 10 repetitions. Two outcomes emerged from this research: first, to produce the same resistance force, the muscle had to be stretched further by 3.5 per cent; and, second, when the muscle was stretched to a pre-set length, the load required to do this gradually reduced. The conclusion is that, over time, the passive resistance offered by muscle to a stretch reduces. Thus static or PNF stretching seems to be more effective than ballistic stretching. In addition, each stretch should be held and the individual stretches repeated for a set of 10 or more repetitions.

Key point:

Both contractile (muscle) and non-contractile (other tissue) factors limit range of motion and provide resistance to movement. With prolonged stretching, the passive resistance produced by a muscle is reduced.

DOES STRETCHING ALTER MUSCLE POWER OUTPUT?

Anyone will recognise that after a hard stretching session the muscles feel shaky and slightly weak. This feeling actually identifies a recognised physiological effect – that of a reduction in strength output following intense stretching. Following hip and knee stretching, Kokkonen et al., (1998) tested subjects with a 1 repetition maximum (1RM) lift. (1RM, or '1 repetition maximum', is the maximum amount of weight that can be lifted in a single repetition.) The subjects' lifting ability was reduced by 7–8 per cent following static stretching.

Using a footplate to stretch and measure strength output from the deep calf (soleus) muscle, Fowles et al., (2000) used 13 maximal passive stretches over a 30-minute period, holding each stretch for over 2 minutes. Again, they measured maximal muscle contraction and found that strength in the stretching group reduced by 28 per cent immediately after stretching, reducing to 12 per cent after 30 minutes and

9 per cent after 60 minutes. Using a leg extension exercise, Behm et al., (2001) used 20 minutes of static stretching, with each repetition held for 45 seconds. These authors found a 12 per cent reduction in maximal leg strength, confirming the results of the previous studies. A number of mechanisms may be responsible for this stretch-induced decline in strength output.

Electrical monitoring of muscle activity (EMG) has revealed a 20 per cent decline in quadriceps activity after stretching (Behm et al., 2001). Stimulating the muscle electrically (a method called interpolated twitch or IT) has also shown decreases in muscle activation of up to 13 per cent (Fowles et al., 2000). We have seen that a variety of muscle reflexes are important to stretching, and it seems that these may contribute to the strength changes. Changes in the stretch reflex and golgi tendon organs have both been proposed as other contributing factors.

Finally, after intense eccentric muscle contraction, there is microscopic damage within the muscle, leading to an increase in a chemical called creatine kinase (CK). Levels of this same chemical are raised by over 60 per cent following intense stretching (Smith et al., 1993), so it seems that muscle damage may also result from performing intense stretching.

So, we can see that prior stretching (stretching before performance) can be detrimental to muscle power output. But, what about strength endurance

Key point:

Intense stretching prior to performance is not recommended, as it will likely result in reduced power output from the muscle. Intense stretching should be an entirely separate part of a training programme.

– that is performing multiple reps rather than a single rep? This is a question answered by Nelson et al., (2005) from Louisiana State University. They had athletes perform strength endurance activities at 60 per cent bodyweight and at 40 per cent bodyweight, with and without prior stretching. Strength endurance was reduced by 24 per cent at 60 per cent bodyweight exercise and by 9 per cent at 40 per cent bodyweight. Both results were statistically significant, and the larger reduction reflects the greater effect of prior stretching on heavier power-based exercise.

The concept of stretching and performance as a whole was addressed by Behm and Chaouachi (2011). They reviewed 42 high-calibre research papers (1606 participants in total) between 1989 and 2011, and showed that a greater number of participants showed a significant impairment in performance. They quoted measures of strength tests, isokinetics, and jump height. From their study these authors identified a variety of sub groups which may be used to guide the prescription of pre-competition stretching (*see* fig 6.1). Shorter-duration static stretches were shown to produce less performance impairment. A maximum stretching volume of 90 seconds (3 reps of 30 seconds each) seems to be a good clinical cut-off, with repetitions of 30 seconds or less leading to very little performance impairment. It should also be noted that performance reductions which are important to competitive athletes may not be significant for those training recreationally. Ranges from no performance reduction on isokinetic torque measurement for a 30-second volume (1 rep of 30-second hold) to a 12.9 per cent reduction for a 300-second volume (20 reps of 15-second hold) have been shown by Zakas et al., (2006). For a recreational athlete, a performance decrement of 5 per cent or less may be tolerable.

The type of performance engaged in following a stretching programme is also important.

Chronic static stretching may have both neural and viscoelastic effects, changing muscle tone and tissue extensibility. Measures such as VO2 max in runners may not be decreased by these changes whereas performance on a vertical jump may be, due to a reduction in storage of elastic energy (*see* chapter 1).

The intensity at which the stretching exercise is practised is also an important variable. Many static stretches are taken to the point of discomfort (POD) to provide the greatest tissue overload. However, taking the stretch to a sub-maximal intensity may reduce performance decrements. A stretching volume of 2 minutes has been shown not to produce a training decrement when a 90 per cent POD was used (Young et al., 2006). Chronic stretching to the POD has been shown

Key point:

To prevent performance decrements when using static stretching, limit both the volume of stretching and its intensity.

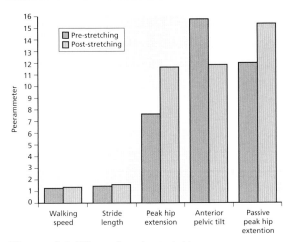

Figure 6.1 Effect of static stretching on performance in 42 scientific studies

to lead to a reduction in EMG and H-reflex activity (Aveda, 1999) demonstrating decreased motoneuron excitation.

CAN STRETCHING IMPROVE PERFORMANCE?

Shrier, a researcher from Quebec, Canada, looked at whether stretching can actually improve performance (Shrier, 2004). Rather than testing individual athletes, Shrier looked at 23 articles which examined the effects of acute stretching (the effect immediately after a stretch has been performed), and nine articles looking at the effects of regular stretching. Analysis of these articles showed that there was no improvement of isometric force, isokinetic torque (individual muscle measures) or jumping height (whole body measure) after acute stretching. Of the nine papers which looked at the long-term effect of stretching, seven papers actually demonstrated improvements in force, jump height and speed.

As opposed to static stretching (hold at full range), dynamic stretching (motion through full range) does not seem to impair subsequent performance, and may actually improve it. Behm and Chaouachi (2011) combined data from a number of studies (241 subjects) to show performance decrement for dynamic stretching of less than 30 seconds' duration, but improvement for 30–90 seconds' duration. Improvement dropped off when dynamic stretching endurance was greater than 90 seconds.

Key point:

Dynamic stretching of 30–90 seconds' duration prior to doing sport may improve performance.

NEURAL STRETCHING

Chapter 13 demonstrates that nerves may be targeted in stretching practice by using specific neural stretch techniques. In the case of the lower back, one of the major nerves to require stretching is the sciatic nerve which runs from the lower back nerve roots, through the buttock and down the back of the thigh. At the back of the lower thigh, the nerve divides into two branches with one (lateral plantar nerve) running to the shin, and the other (tibial nerve) running on into the foot and toes. To stretch the nerve we can use the slump stretch, which is a modification of a physiotherapy test used to assess the nerve itself. The slump combines a straight leg and dorsiflexed foot to stretch the lower part of the nerve, with trunk and neck flexion to stretch the top portion. The arms are held behind the back (hands clasped) to place tension on the nerve sheaths of the upper body, remembering that the nerve sheaths of the upper limb, spinal cord, and lower limb are all linked.

Cleland et al., (2006) used a slump stretch with low back pain patients who had mild symptoms. Subjects were assessed using self-report pain measures and a disability index questionnaire (Oswestry Disability Index or ODI). They completed a slump stretch programme, sitting

Definition:

Centralisation is a phenomenon seen during the recovery of low back pain with referred pain, normally into the leg. Those with severe conditions may have pain referring through the whole leg and into the foot. As the symptoms subside, they appear further up the leg to the calf or knee, and eventually centralise into the buttock and, finally, back into the spine.

Slump position with feet against wall, hands clasped behind back. Therapist applies overpressure to whole spine flexion. Stretch stopped at point of symptoms onset and held for 30s.

Home exercise providing overpressure using hands behind head. Stretch stopped at point of symptoms onset and held for 30s.

Figure 6.2a and **b** Slump stretching

with their legs straight, ankles dorsiflexed (0 degrees) and feet flat against a wall. Overpressure was applied to the cervical spine by the therapist to the point at which the subject's symptoms were produced (*see* fig 6.2(a)). The position was held for 30 seconds, and 5 repetitions were performed over a period of 3–4 minutes. Patients performed a slump stretch using self-applied overpressure (hands behind head) as home exercise (*see* fig 6.2(b)). At the end of the study, those who had practised the slump stretch demonstrated statistically significant improvement of disability score, pain reduction and symptom centralisation.

STRETCHING IN THE ELDERLY

Increased falling in the elderly is associated with changes in a number of fitness components (S Factors, chapter 4). Reduction in strength and muscle mass due to ageing (sarcopaenia) is often considered important clinically, as is a reduction in balance ability – frequently measured in the clinic using Romberg's test to assess standing balance.

Falling during locomotion (walking, turning, stair climbing for example) has been shown to be influenced by a number of gait parameters, with a reduction in hip extension range shown

to be most relevant. Rodackia et al., (2009) used a single stretching session targeting the hip flexor musculature with a modified Thomas test (chapter 5) using 4 repetitions of a 60-second hold (static stretch). Analysis of subjects' gait pattern following stretching demonstrated a greater step length, which with unchanged cadence gave a 6.6 per cent increase in walking velocity. Change in walking velocity is important because gait speed has been shown to be one of the most important predictors of falling in the elderly (Dargent-Molina, 1996). Increases in both anterior pelvic tilt and pelvic rotation in the transverse plane were also shown. A shorter stance time was also seen with a reduced double leg support and increased swing duration. The increased time in support led to improved balance. Although stretching effects following a single exercise session are unlikely to be maintained, they do create a therapy window in which to re-educate gait, and a period of pain and risk reduction if used as part of a home exercise programme. In addition, the effect of stretching on important gait parameters is illustrated, justifying the use of hip flexor stretching for fall prevention in the elderly. Watt et al., (2011) used a supervised hip flexor stretching programme over 10 weeks to change gait parameters in subjects over 65 years of age. They used a half-lunge exercise (*see* page 115) in 82 healthy subjects, dividing the group into those who received the hip flexor stretch, and a control group who received a shoulder stretching exercise instead. Each group performed 2 sets of their stretching exercise (on both the right and left sides of the body) each held for 60 seconds, daily. The hip stretching group showed statistically significant increases in passive hip extension range, increased stride length, peak hip extension, and decreased anterior pelvic tilt after the programme. In contrast, the control group did not show the same improvements (*see* fig 6.3).

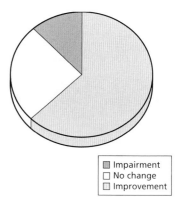

☐ Impairment
☐ No change
☐ Improvement

Figure 6.3 Effects on a hip-stretching programme on gait in the elderly

Key point:

Stretching is important in seniors and can lead to positive changes in gait pattern.

STRETCHING FOR RESPIRATORY CONDITIONS

Chronic respiratory conditions often result in a loss of compliance (give or springiness) of the chest structures. The relatively fixed position of the ribs results in a barrel chest appearance with wasting of the intercostal muscles and the diaphragm. Stretching exercise has been successfully used in the treatment of respiratory conditions. Leelarungrayub et al., (2009) used chest wall and thoracic stretching (thoracic rotation, mid-sternum compression and lateral thoracic stretching in sitting together with lateral thoracic stretching performed over pillows

Definition:

(i) *Expired tidal volume* is the volume of air breathed out of the lungs in quiet respiration and is a measured (objective) value. (ii) *Dyspnea* is shortness of breath (breathlessness) and is an experience felt by the patient (subjective). (iii) *COPD* is a chronic lung condition where the respiratory airways are restricted or blocked. The condition is commonly due to lung tissue inflammation and breakdown caused by tobacco smoking and/or environmental factors.

in side lying) for 10 minutes daily for 5 days in a 60-year-old patient with chronic obstructive pulmonary disease (COPD). The results showed a significant clinical improvement of expired tidal volume (measured using a respirometer), reduction in dyspnea level (measured using a Borg scale), and increase in chest expansion (recorded using a tape measure of chest circumference) following stretching.

Chronic respiratory conditions frequently result in secondary changes to the shoulder and neck muscles with the pectoral muscles and anterior scalenes in particular often being tight. Changes to these muscles exacerbate dyspnea as they are secondary muscles of respiration which assist in chest expansion in times of laboured breathing. In addition, changes to the muscles result in postural alteration and reduction of functional usage of the upper limb. Stretching of the shoulder musculature has been shown to be effective in patients with chronic respiratory conditions, improving both shoulder movement range and function. Putt et al., (2008) used contract relaxed stretching exercise in sitting (90 degree shoulder abduction, glenohumeral rotation resisted) in a double blind crossover trial of 14 patients with COPD. When compared to a sham intervention, patients who received the stretching programme showed a statistically significant improvement in shoulder motion range and vital capacity, a lung measure of the maximum amount of air which can be breathed out (exhaled) after a full breath in (inspiration). The results clearly demonstrated the effect of stretching on both shoulder and respiratory function.

Key point:

Stretching exercises targeting the ribcage and thoracic spine are useful in treating those with chronic chest conditions.

STRETCHING AS RELAXATION TRAINING

Many common forms of relaxation training such as progressive relaxation, aim to facilitate physical relaxation by reducing resting muscle tone. Physical relaxation of this types is thought to encourage mental relaxation demonstrating

the popular mind-body nature of exercise types such as yoga. Progressive relaxation involves isometric contraction of the target muscle (typically for 5–7 seconds) followed by muscle release/relaxation for 20–30 seconds. One of the underlying principles of progressive relaxation is that of post-isometric relaxation which relies on activation of golgi tendon organs (GTO, see chapter 3). Static stretching will also activate the GTO and can lead to a reduction in muscle tone following its practice, making the use of static stretching potentially suitable as a relaxation procedure. Carlson et al., (1990) used a set of stretching exercises (10-second hold) to reduce muscle tone in four muscle groups (obicularis oculi, trapezius, biceps, sternocleidomastoid and forearm flexors). They showed a statistically significant reduction in muscle tone and self-reported anxiety measures.

Tight muscles often develop painful trigger points and this is especially the case in the muscles around the neck and shoulders including the trapezius, levator scapulae, rhomboids, and scalenes. The combination of PNF stretching and trigger point release manual therapy has been shown to be effective in the release of painful trigger points (Trampasa et al., 2010). The short-term gains in movement range in this type of treatment are thought to result from sarcomere release (give) and an analgesic effect produced by stretching.

The relationship between muscle tension measured on EMG and anxiety score is underlined by Engel and Andersen (2000), in a mind-body study with patients which combined mindful (meditative) stretching with body awareness training. Body awareness training was practised in supine lying using breath control to focus attention on different parts of the body in turn. Meditative stretching consisted of 14 stretching exercises linked in a sequence which lasted for

20 minutes. Each stretch position was moved into on an out breath and held for 3–4 breaths (static stretch). EMG of the frontalis muscle of the forehead decreased by 31 per cent, and state anxiety by 22 per cent. Alpha brain wave activity (a measure of relaxation and meditation) increased by 52 per cent during the exercise period.

Key point:

Stretching exercises can be used as part of a relaxation programme.

SUMMARY

- The angle of pelvic tilt is important for the application of stretches around the hip, especially for the hamstrings.
- Stretching reduces the 'stiffness' in a muscle in much the same way as a warm-up does. Over time, this may have a protective effect on the muscle-tendon unit in many power-based activities.
- Tendon, ligaments, nerves and the joint capsule will also limit the range of motion at a joint.
- Ice may be used to reduce muscle spasm prior to stretching.
- Following intense stretching, the power output of a muscle can be reduced.
- Combining heat with stretching will give better results than warming prior to stretching.
- Muscle reflexes are important to the stretching process.
- A 30-second static stretch is most effective, and 4–5 repetitions only should be applied.
- To prevent performance decrements when using static stretching, limit both the volume of stretching and its intensity.
- Intense stretching immediately before competitive sport is not recommended.
- Stretching can favourably change gait patterns in the elderly.
- Stretching may be used in both respiratory conditions and to aid muscle relaxation.

PART TWO

THE EXERCISES

BEGINNER STRETCHES

7

INTRODUCTION TO THE STRETCHING EXERCISES

In this chapter we begin to look at a variety of stretching exercises. The list is by no means exhaustive, but it includes the most useful exercises for sport, health and therapy. The exercises are loosely grouped into sections, each under a separate chapter number. The beginner, intermediate and advanced stretch groupings take into account the complexity of the movement, and the difficulty of performing the exercises with good alignment. However, any movement may become an advanced stretch simply by pressing into a greater range of motion. Within each of these chapters the order of the exercises is based on three main areas of the body: upper limbs, trunk and lower limbs, respectively. Tables 7.1(a), 7.1(b) and 7.1(c) provide details of the muscles stretched for each exercise movement for each of these areas of the body. There are also chapters showing stretches for the nerves (neural stretches), linked tissues (fascial stretches), partner stretches and stretches that a therapist or personal trainer may apply to a client. In the final chapter we will look at some common yoga exercises and see the similarities and differences to stretching actions.

Before performing any of the movements, make sure that you are thoroughly warmed up; you should be sweating lightly and wrapped in loose-fitting clothing to maintain body heat. All exercises should be performed slowly, encouraging, rather than forcing, the action. The stretch should be placed on the muscle when exhaling, and the final position held for 20–30 seconds, while breathing normally. You should feel a comfortable stretch, but no pain.

Starting position and instructions refer to the right-hand side of the body, but can be applied to the left-hand side just as easily. 'Lie on the floor' will always refer to lying on your back, unless otherwise stated.

Variations of exercises are included because these prevent you from getting stale. In addition, two or three exercises designed to stretch exactly the same muscles will each stress the body in slightly different ways. These different stresses reduce the likelihood of you developing overuse injuries. You will have preferences for certain exercises, and some will suit you more than others do, depending on your body size and make-up. This is fine, and serves to individualise your stretching programme.

Points to note are important because these are sometimes concerned with safety factors and injury prevention. You may like to make a note of any points you find relevant to your own training style after reading this section on an exercise.

The following are also useful references: figure 1.15 Anatomical terminology (*see* page 19), figure 1.14 Axes and planes (*see* page 18), and table 4.5 Starting positions (*see* page 63).

Table 7.1(a)	Upper limbs
Joint movement	**Muscles stretched**
Shoulder protraction	Rhomboid major, rhomboid minor, trapezius
Shoulder retraction	Serratus anterior, pectoralis minor
Shoulder depression	Trapezius (upper fibres), levator scapulae
Shoulder adduction	Suprasinatus, deltoid
Shoulder extension	Pectoralis major, deltoid (anterior fibres), biceps brachii (long head), coracobrachialis
Shoulder flexion	Latissimus dorsi, teres major, pectoralis major, deltoid (posterior fibres), triceps (long head)
Shoulder abduction	Coracobrachialis, pectoralis major, latissimus dorsi, teres major
Shoulder lateral rotation	Subscapularis, teres major, latissimus dorsi, pectoralis major, deltoid (anterior fibres)
Shoulder medial rotation	Teres minor, infraspinatus, deltoid (posterior fibres)
Elbow extension	Biceps brachii, brachialis, brachioradialis, pronator teres
Elbow flexion	Triceps brachii, anconeus
Forearm supination	Pronator teres, pronator quadratus, brachiordialis
Wrist extension	Flexor carpi ulnaris, flexor carpi radialis, Palmaris longus, flexor digitorum superficialis, flexor digitorum profundus, flexor pollicis longus
Wrist flexion	Extensor carpi radialis longus, extensor carpi radialis brevis, extensor carpi ulnaris, extensor digitorum, extensor indicis, extensor digiti minimi, extensor pollicis longus, extensor pollicis brevis

Table 7.1(b)	Trunk
Joint movement	**Muscles stretched**
Extension	Rectus abdominis, external oblique, internal oblique, psoas minor, psoas major
Rotation	Multifidus, rotatores, semispinalis, internal oblique, external oblique
Lateral flexion	Quadratus lumborum, intertransversarii, external oblique, internal oblique, rectus abdominis, erector spinae, multifidus
Flexion	Quadratus lumborum, multifidus, semispinalis, erector spinae, interspinales

Table 7.1(c)	Lower limbs
Joint movement	**Muscles stretched**
Hip flexion	Gluteus maximus, hamstrings (semiendinosus, semimembranosus, biceps femoris)
Hip adduction	Gluteus maximus, gluteus medius, gluteus minimus, tensor fascia lata
Hip abduction	Adductor magnus, adductor longus, adductor brevis, gracilis, pectineus
Hip extension	Psoas major, iliacus, rectus femoris, sartorius, pectineus
Hip lateral (outward) rotation	Anterior part of gluteus medius, anterior part of gluteus minimus, tensor fascia lata, psoas major, iliacus
Hip medial (inward) rotation	Gluteus maximus, piriformis, obturator internus, gemellus superior, gemellus inferior, quadratus femoris, obturator externus
Knee joint extension	Hamstrings (semitendinosus, semimembranosus, biceps femoris), gastrocnemius, gracilis, sartorius
Knee joint flexion	Quadriceps femoris (rectus femoris, vastus lateralis, vastus intermedius, vastus medialis), tensor fascia lata
Ankle joint dorsiflexion	Gastrocnemius, soleus, plantaris, peroneus longus, tibialis posterior, flexor digitorum longus, flexor hallucis longus
Ankle joint plantarflexion	Tibialis anterior, extensor digitorum longus, extensor hallucis longus, peroneus tertius

BUILDING A STRETCHING PROGRAMME

There is a number of reasons that a person begins to use stretching exercise. You might be an athlete with a full training regime simply wanting to integrate a few stretching exercises into your current programme, or an office worker looking to use stretches to counteract day-to-day stiffness. Some people will want to use stretching as a therapy to regain lost movement following an injury, while others may simply want to improve their posture. Whatever your reason for embarking upon a stretching programme, you need to decide which of the exercises are most appropriate for your needs. The herd instinct is ever-present in sport, and people often perform the same stretches as their friend or teammates.

Although this is understandable, each person has very different needs. If you have tight shoulders and long hamstrings but your training partner has very short hamstrings, performing the same exercises does not make sense. One person could easily struggle with an exercise while the other finds it so easy as not to be challenging. Identify your stretching needs and structure a personalised programme accordingly. Let's look briefly at how to build a stretching programme by putting a variety of exercises together.

If you are completely new to exercise it is often useful to work with a personal trainer to learn exercise technique. This can be important because as an inexperienced user it is often difficult to recognise when a technique is poor. If you practise an exercise thinking you are using it correctly

Key point:

Spend time to identify your needs and choose stretches for your requirements. Do not simply perform the same stretches as a friend or training partner.

when in fact your alignment is poor you simply rehearse the poor movement which then becomes a habit, and difficult to correct. A personal trainer is able to look at your alignment from outside your body and correct you accordingly. Investing in a few sessions at the beginning of your stretching career can put you on the right track to ensure that you practise an exercise correctly from now on.

We have seen that the first part of the programme is a warm-up which aims to induce light sweating. This will increase the blood flow to the muscles to be stretched and in so doing warm the tissues, making them more malleable. In addition, it can act as a psychological break between your 'office mindset' and that of exercise. If you have performed another type of exercise immediately before you stretch, your body may already be warm and so the aim now is to relax your body and reduce muscle tone prior to stretching. So, the warm-up acts as a preparation for stretching and may either increase or decrease your body's 'tick over' (metabolic rate) depending on your prior condition.

Once the body has been prepared for stretching we choose exercises for the arms, legs and trunk to balance the programme. In order to keep blood in the region which is working it is useful to put several exercises for a body part together. So, for example, if we choose three leg stretches within a programme these would be practised one after another rather than separated. This is in contrast to circuit training for the cardiovascular system where arms, legs and trunk are alternated to keep the heart rate high while at the same time reducing fatigue on the working muscles. When we use a number of stretches on one body area such as the leg we begin with the larger muscle groups (hip) and move on to the smaller muscle groups (knee and shin). This is because smaller muscle groups fatigue more quickly and can act as a limiting factor to other stretches.

For a general stretching programme, aim to incorporate at least one exercise for each of the main body parts, that is the upper and lower spine, the hip and knee, the shoulder and elbow. You may find that one exercise works several body parts. For example, *hamstrings stretch – long sitting* (exercise 3) works the hamstrings at the hip and knee, together with the whole spine moving into flexion. Other movements may isolate a body part and in so doing can avoid excessive movement at another area which may not be wanted. For example, *knee extension – with towel* (*see* page 176) again works the hamstrings at the hip and knee, but eliminates movement at the lower back.

For a general stretching programme, begin with static stretches, holding each stretch for 10–20 seconds and breathing normally. When you want to increase the intensity of the stretch, hold for a longer period (30–40 seconds) and pull into the position more firmly. A stretching exercise will give an intense sensation within the muscle being lengthened. This can be scored on a visual analogue scale (VAS) from 0 to 10 (*see* fig 7.1). When you begin a programme hold the stretch at a fairly low intensity (0 to 4) and as you progress the exercise increase the holding intensity (5 to 8). Ensure when you perform the static stretch that you don't hold your breath; aim to breathe normally allowing the breath to flow evenly and not breathing too often or too deeply (hyperventilating).

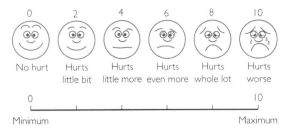

No hurt | Hurts little bit | Hurts little more | Hurts even more | Hurts whole lot | Hurts worse

Figure 7.1 Visual analogue scale

Definition:

Hyperventilation occurs when you breathe too quickly or deeply and remove too much carbon dioxide from your bloodstream. This upsets the balance between acid and alkali in the blood resulting in alkalosis (rise in pH value). Symptoms include dizziness, tingling in the hands and feet, and fainting.

If you are new to stretching aim to progress through the beginner, intermediate and advanced stretches. Each stage should take you between 4 to 8 weeks, but allow additional time if you have problems with a particular body part. If you are familiar with exercise you may start with any movement which suits your requirements. Where you have particular issues with posture look at the modified stretches in the posture section, and where you have clinical conditions read the chapters on stretching for nerves, fascia and injuries. For those wanting to enhance sporting performance the dynamic and partner stretches may be useful. However, it is always better to begin with a sound foundation provided by the beginner and intermediate stretches before using the more complex or intense movements.

Exercise 1 Hip adductors – long sitting

Starting position and instructions

Sit on the floor with both legs straight. Flex your right leg, placing your foot on your left thigh above the knee. Support the foot with your left hand, and press down on the knee with your right hand. Lengthen your spine and maintain spinal alignment throughout the movement.

Variations

Start by sitting with your back flat against a wall and a rolled towel placed in the small of your back (lumbar area) to maintain spinal alignment. You can sit on a wedge to anteriorly tilt the pelvis. If your knee is too stiff to bend so that your foot rests on your thigh, rest your foot just below the knee, on the shin.

Points to note

Most individuals are asymmetrical and will find that one leg is more flexible than the other. There is a tendency with this exercise for those who have reduced flexibility of the adductors to tilt the body towards the bent knee, lifting the pelvis and buttock (ischial) from the floor. This gives an apparent increase in flexibility as the knee can be lowered further, but there is no greater stretch placed on the adductors.

Exercise 2 Gluteal stretch – lying

Starting position and instructions

Lie on the floor with the left leg straight. Flex the right knee and pull it upwards and across towards the left shoulder.

Variations

Pulling the knee across the body rather than towards the shoulder will vary the emphasis of the stretch.

Points to note

This exercise also places stress on the pelvis, so it is inappropriate after pregnancy. Also, the combination of extreme hip flexion and adduction makes the exercise dangerous to those who have had a hip replacement operation.

Exercise 3 Hamstrings stretch – long sitting

Starting position and instructions

Sit with your left leg straight and your right leg comfortably bent. Reach forwards with the left hand to grip your left foot. Press your right hand on your left knee to maintain knee extension. Maintain spinal alignment, gently curving throughout the whole spine.

Variations

Place both hands on the left knee, lengthen your spine and hinge only from the hip avoiding spinal flexion. Alternatively, loop a belt or towel under your foot and pull on the belt rather than on the foot directly. Placing the belt under the ball of the foot and toes rather than the heel will cause an additional stretch on the tissue that forms the sole of the foot (plantar fascia).

Points to note

Individuals who are hyperflexible in the thoracic spine may place excessive stress on this area. To avoid this, retract the shoulders, expand the chest and maintain this position throughout the exercise. If you find you are still unable to maintain your spinal alignment, reverse the order of the exercise to change the emphasis. Begin with your knee unlocked (slightly bent) and reach forwards with a straight spine. Once in the stretched position, attempt to straighten the leg.

Exercise 4 Hamstrings – active knee extension

Starting position and instructions
Lie on the floor with the left leg straight and flex the right knee and hip to 90 degrees. Grip your hands behind the right knee and actively straighten the leg using your quadriceps muscles. The knee should remain directly above the hip.

Variations
Place your hand on the front of the leg and actively push your leg on to your hand using the power of your hip flexors; at the same time, extend your knee. This will cause the hamstring muscles to further relax through reflex action.

Points to note
Pulling the toes towards you and flexing your neck will throw stress on to the neural tissues and sciatic nerve and away from the hamstrings (*see* Stretching the nerves, chapter 13).

Exercise 5 Hamstrings stretch – supported by a door frame

Starting position and instructions
Start by lying on the floor in a doorway. Your hips should be level with the door frame. Bend your left leg and place your left foot on the upright of the frame, keeping your right leg straight on the ground. Straighten your left leg, sliding your left heel up the door frame as you do so.

Variations
Moving your whole body forwards or backwards so that the door frame is at waist or knee level will cause a greater or lesser amount of hip flexion and change the intensity of the exercise.

Points to note
Make sure that your heel stays on the door frame to take the weight of your leg. If you find that your foot does not slide readily, keep your sock on to increase slip.

Exercise 6 Rectus femoris stretch – standing

Starting position and instructions

Stand side-on to a wall with your right hand supporting your bodyweight. Flex your left leg and grip your ankle with your knee flexed. Pull your left hip back into extension, while maintaining correct spinal alignment.

Variations

Loop a towel around your ankle to reduce the amount of knee flexion and to allow you to pull in to further hip extension, which will emphasise the upper portion of the muscle.

Points to note

This exercise also stretches the femoral nerve (*see* page 196). A sensation of burning or tingling (pins and needles) over the front of the thigh suggests that this nerve may be tight or possibly trapped, requiring physiotherapy management.

Exercise 7 Calf stretch – wall lean

Starting position and instructions

Stand facing a wall with both feet together, arms straight and hands on the wall. Keeping your legs straight, bend your arms to lower your trunk towards the wall.

Variations

Walking towards or away from the wall will change the emphasis of the exercise.

Points to note

Asymmetry is common in this area, so you may find that one arm can bend more than the other. This movement stretches the superficial calf muscle, the gastrocnemius.

Exercise 8 Calf lunge

Starting position and instructions

Begin by facing a wall in a half-lunge position with your left foot forward. Place your hands on the wall and bend your arms to lower your bodyweight forwards, pressing your left foot into dorsiflexion.

Variations

Altering the angle of the foot away from the perpendicular will change the emphasis on the calf muscle.

Points to note

The heel must remain on the floor throughout the movement. As the knee is bent in this movement, the stretch on the superficial calf muscle (gastrocnemius) is reduced and that on the deep calf muscle (soleus) increased.

Exercise 9 Sit back on heels

Starting position and instructions

Begin kneeling on all fours (4-point kneeling) on a mat or folded towel. Move your hips backwards over your ankles and press your shins and tops of your feet (dorum) to the ground. Keep your feet and shin parallel so you get an even stretch across your foot.

Variations

Sit back turning your feet inwards or outwards to vary the stretch effect. To increase the stretch intensity, take more of your bodyweight on to your shins by releasing your hands and sitting up to take your weight on your knees alone (2-point kneeling). This action then becomes the anterior tibialis stretch (exercise 18).

Points to note

This action presses the foot into plantarflexion to stretch the shin muscles (tibialis anterior especially). However, the ankle joint is also stretched, and if you have a very stiff ankle following a sprain or fracture you may need to place a folded towel between your shin and the floor to reduce the movement range at your ankle.

Exercise 10 Spinal rotation – on a chair

Exercise 11 Lower back flexion – lying

Starting position and instructions

Begin sitting side-on to a firm-backed chair. Turn towards the chair back and grasp the top of the backrest frame keeping your elbows apart. Use your hands to gently press further into rotation. Release the action and turn around, rotating the spine in the opposite direction, in each case towards the chair back.

Variations

Sit diagonally across the chair with the side of the backrest pressed against your tailbone (sacrum). Turn towards the chair back as above – the altered sitting angle increases the movement range.

Points to note

As you turn keep your shoulder level, do not dip to one side. Any dipping action will impose side flexion with the rotation action closing the facet joints on the convex side of the spine.

Starting position and instructions

Lie on the floor, drawing your knees up to your chest. Grip your knees and pull them into your chest and up towards your shoulders, creating a rocking position in your lower spine. This movement stretches the erector spinae.

Variations

This movement can be combined with rotation or lateral flexion to alter the stress on your spine.

Points to note

The movement is one of pulling your knees towards your shoulders rather than pulling your knees in towards your chest.

Exercise 12 Whole back flexion – sitting

Starting position and instructions

Begin by sitting on a stool or firm chair with your hips slightly above your knees and your feet hip width apart. Place your hands on your thighs to take some of the weight of your trunk throughout the movement. Start the movement by bending your neck and pulling your chin down to your chest. Continue the action by flexing your thoracic spine, aiming your nose towards your umbilicus, and finally allow the lumbar spine to bend as though bringing your head between your knees. Pause in the lower position and then straighten your spine, section by section, until you are sitting upright again.

Variations

You can emphasise different sections of your spine with this movement. Beginning with neck flexion initiates movement at the upper thoracic spine, while keeping the neck in line with the rest of the spine throws the stretch to the mid- and lower thoracic spine. As you bend forwards, tucking the tail under (posterior pelvic tilt) throws the emphasis lower down the lumbar spine.

Points to note

Make sure that you begin the exercise by taking most of your upper bodyweight through your hands. As you become more confident with the movement, you can change the exercise into more of a controlled strength action by releasing the arms and allowing them to hang at the sides of the knees. In this way, you control the action using an eccentric (muscle lengthening) action of the spinal extensors going down and a concentric (muscle shortening) action as you come back up.

The action should feel as though your spine is a column of bricks; as you bend, you are moving one brick at a time, unstacking and then stacking the vertebrae back up again.

Exercise 13 Thoracic spine – kneeling

Starting position and instructions

Kneeling on all fours, sit back on your ankles, keeping your hands fixed. Feel the stretch in the latissimus dorsi muscle and thoracolumbar fascia and the thoracic spine.

Variations

Placing one knee slightly forwards of the other will impart some lateral flexion on your spine.

Points to note

This position may be held for 30–120 seconds to gain full benefit of the stretch on your spine.

Exercise 14 Thoracic spine – sitting

Starting position and instructions

Begin by sitting on a high backed chair with a towel folded over the top of the chair back for padding. Sit right back in the chair so that your buttocks actually contact the chair back. Extend your thoracic spine over the back of the chair using the padded upper edge as a pivot point. Draw your elbows and upper arms backwards to supply force for the stretch.

Variations

The exact point at which the stretch is felt will depend on the contact point between the upper edge of the chair back and the thoracic spine. Shuttling up and down to place the chair edge higher or lower on the spine will vary the emphasis of the stretch.

Points to note

As you extend the thoracic spine backwards, make sure that your hips do not simply slide forwards, as this will release part of the stretch, reducing its effectiveness. As you extend the thoracic spine, the ribcage will be expanded, so breathe in as you stretch and out as you release it.

Exercise 15 Shoulder rotation

Starting position and instructions

Kneel and internally rotate and extend the shoulders to place both of your hands behind you on the small of your back. Draw your elbows back and together to stretch the external rotators and flexors of the shoulder (teres minor, supraspinatus, infraspinatus, deltoid and long head of the biceps muscles).

Variations

Moving the hands up towards the shoulders, or down towards the knees, will vary the site of the stretch.

Points to note

Optimal spinal alignment must be maintained throughout this exercise. The lumbar spine must not be hyperextended.

Exercise 16 Tricep stretch – standing

Starting position and instructions

Stand with your feet hip width apart. Reach overhead with your left arm and bend the elbow so that your left hand touches your back behind your left shoulder. Reach up with your right hand and grip your left elbow, pressing the left arm towards the vertical.

Variations

Bending the elbow less far (to 90 degrees rather than to full extension) will take some of the stretch away from the lower portion of the triceps and throw proportionally more stretch on to the upper portion. This is because the triceps is a two-joint (biarticular) muscle with actions over both the shoulder and the elbow.

Points to note

If you find that you have a tendency to lean backwards as you press your elbow overhead, perform the exercise sitting on a gym bench to aid the maintenance of spinal alignment.

INTERMEDIATE STRETCHES

8

Exercise 17 Calf and Achilles – prolonged stretch

Starting position and instructions
Stand with your back against a wall and your feet about 10 cm in front of your body-line. Place your toes and forefeet on a small (2 cm-high) block or book and allow your heels to rest on the floor. Rest your body against the wall and maintain the position for 5–10 minutes.

Variations
Choosing a thicker block increases the stretch, while a thinner one reduces it. In each case, it is important that the heel rests on the floor throughout the exercise.

Points to note
This exercise offers a prolonged low-level stretch on the calf and Achilles. Because the heel rests on the floor, the calf muscles are able to relax instead of having to hold the position through an eccentric contraction. The combination of muscle relaxation and the length of time the stretch is held for makes this movement suitable for stretching after injury where swelling has built up and clotted to form tough scar tissue within the muscle or tendon.

Exercise 18 Anterior tibialis

Exercise 19 Hip flexors – Thomas test position

Starting position and instructions

Kneel on the floor and then sit back on your ankles, pressing the front of the ankles to the floor.

Variations

Place a folded towel beneath your toes to press them into flexion and increase the stretch on the toe extensors.

Points to note

This exercise places considerable stress on the knees. People with knee pain should perform the exercise while leaning on a stool to support their bodyweight.

Starting position and instructions

Lie on a bench with your right leg over the bench end. Flex your left hip and knee and pull your knee towards your chest.

Variations

Start with both knees bent and the feet flat on the bench. Pull one knee to the chest and then lower the opposite leg.

Points to note

This is a basic clinical test of hip flexor tightness in the iliopsoas and rectus femoris of the lower leg: increasing the flexion at the knee emphasises the rectus femoris; reducing the knee flexion (straightening the leg) emphasises the iliopsoas.

Exercise 20 Hip flexors – half-lunge position

Starting position and instructions
Kneel on your right leg with your left leg out in front of you and tighten your abdominal muscles to stabilise your trunk. Press your left leg forwards, forcing your left hip into extension.

Variations
Support your weight with one hand on a stool, or place your left forearm along the length of your left thigh. If you find yourself tending to lose spinal alignment, reach your right arm overhead as though you are trying to touch the ceiling; lengthening the entire body will help to emphasise good spinal alignment.

Points to note
Altering the degree of hip rotation will change the emphasis on the hip flexors. Relaxing the abdominal muscles and allowing the pelvis to tilt forwards will give the impression of a greater range of motion at the hip, but will actually stress the lumbar spine.

Exercise 21 Bilateral hip adductors – sitting

Starting position and instructions
Sit on the floor and place the soles of your feet together. Grip your feet and press down on your knees or thighs using your elbows. Maintain spinal alignment and try to lengthen your spine, reaching your head towards the ceiling as you press down with your elbows. Do not allow your pelvis to tilt backwards.

Variations
Sit on a wedge so that your pelvis is tilted forwards and your spine maintains its lumbar lordosis.

Points to note
Because the adductor muscles are attached to the pubic bone there is a tendency with this exercise to tilt the pelvis backwards and bring the pubic bone forwards, releasing the stretch from the muscle. When this is done the knee will lower further, but there is no greater stretch placed on the adductors. Maintaining the lumbar lordosis and the neutral pelvic position is therefore essential.

Exercise 22 Short adductor wall stretch

Exercise 23 Hip adductors – wide splits

Starting position and instructions

Lie on the floor with your legs straight up and your buttocks close to the wall. Bend your knees and place the soles of your feet together with the sides of your feet resting on the wall itself. Place your hands over your knees and gently press your knees down towards the wall.

Variations

You may keep one leg straight, and place the foot of your bent knee on the straight leg thigh mimicking the position of exercise 1 (*see* page 104).

Points to note

This exercise is similar to exercise 21, but with the whole body rotated through 90 degrees. Now, instead of the legs being supported on the floor allowing the back to bend, the back is kept straight throughout the movement. If you find your arms are not long enough to reach to your knees without flexing your spine, use two small blocks (yoga bricks) placed on your thighs to 'lengthen your arms'.

Starting position and instructions

Sit on the floor. Adduct your hips and place your hands on the floor behind your trunk. Press down with the hands to push the hips forwards, anteriorly tilting your pelvis to increase the stretch.

Variations

Sit with your back flat on the wall and flex and extend your feet to work your ankles further apart.

Points to note

Make sure the ankles do not slide forwards, releasing the adductor stretch.

Exercise 24 Hip adductors – wall support

Starting position and instructions

Lie on the floor with your legs straight up in the air and your buttocks close to a wall. Rest your legs against the wall and allow them to lower slowly out to the sides and downwards into hip abduction. Hold this position for 20–30 seconds and then bring the legs back up again by 20–30 cm (resisted adduction), before again allowing them to lower.

Variations

Lifting the legs against their own weight provides resistance for contract–relax (CR) stretching. This can be increased by having your training partner resist the adduction movement for you by pressing down on your legs.

Points to note

Although this is a stretching exercise, the legs are lowered by an eccentric contraction of the hip adductor muscles and then held in place by an isometric contraction of the same muscles. As the hip adductors relax, movement is increased. The exercise therefore serves to aid adductor muscle relaxation, reducing muscle tone.

Exercise 25 Gluteals on a bench

Starting position and instructions

Begin standing facing a high gym bench or table top. Bend your left leg and place your left foot on the bench. Allow your left knee to lower down to bench level so your hip is flexed and externally rotated. Gently press your knee down to increase the stretch intensity.

Variations

Move your foot out to the side or inwards slightly to vary the stretch emphasis.

Points to note

As you are standing on one leg when performing this stretch make sure that you are stable by holding on to the bench or table. Use a bench height which is comfortable for you and does not tip you off balance.

Exercise 26 Hamstrings and spine – sit and reach position

Exercise 27 Hamstrings – standing

Starting position and instructions

Sit on the floor with your legs straight out in front of you. Reach forwards to touch your toes, curling evenly through the whole of your spine. This exercise stretches the hamstrings and the spine. If an individual is hyperflexible in the thoracic spine, this area will take an excessive stretch. Spinal alignment must be maintained throughout the exercise.

Variations

Start the exercise in the same position with a straight spine, press the chest forwards and retract the shoulders. Move only from the hips using a hinge action. Alternatively, start the exercise with your legs bent and reach forwards as far as you can. Hold this position as you try to straighten first one and then the other leg.

Points to note

The first modification reduces the forwards distance you reach, but increases the stretch on the hamstrings. The second modification reduces the momentum caused by moving the heavy trunk forwards and focuses the stretch more precisely on the hamstrings.

Starting position and instructions

Stand with your feet hip width apart and your knees slightly bent. Bend forwards, keeping your spine as straight as possible so that you move from the hip rather than through the spine. Bend your knee so that you can press your chest against your thighs. Reach around your calves and grip your shins or ankles then, keeping your chest on your knees, try to straighten your legs. Stop at the point where your chest begins to lift from your thighs and hold the position for 20–30 seconds.

Variations

You can practise the same movement sitting on a mat or in a chair. In each case, the movement begins with the chest on the thighs and the aim is to straighten the legs up to the point where the chest begins to lift from the thighs. Hold this position for 20–30 seconds.

Points to note

The standing position is not suitable if you have a history of low-back pain, as it places significant leverage forces on the lumbar region. Choose one of the sitting positions instead. If you find the leg straightening action too intense, hold just one leg straight first and then the other.

Exercise 28 Hamstrings – flat back stretch

Starting position and instructions

Stand in front of a waist-high object or as close as you can such as a low cupboard or piece of gym equipment with your feet hip width apart and your legs straight. Keeping your trunk very straight, bend forwards at the hips and reach your arms out to rest on the ledge in front of you. Make sure that your hips, shoulders, elbows and hands form a straight line.

Variations

Instead of supporting yourself on a ledge, you can place your hands on your knees or thighs and support your bodyweight in the flat back position through your locked arms.

Points to note

The aim of this movement is to place a stretch on the hamstrings by tilting the pelvis forwards and keeping the spine straight or even slightly hollow (lumbar lordosis maintained). To facilitate this, pull your abdomen in and slightly brace your shoulders while pressing your chest outwards (thoracic extension).

Exercise 29 Hamstrings – sitting

Starting position and instructions

Sit on a bench or stool that allows you to reach the floor with your right leg straight and your left leg bent. Tilt your pelvis forwards and, keeping your spine straight, reach forwards towards your knees. Support your bodyweight through your arms throughout the exercise.

Variations

Pulling the foot and toes up towards you and flexing the neck and spine will increase the emphasis on the neural tissues and sciatic nerve.

Points to note

Those who have had back pain may have tightness in the neural tissues or sciatic nerve, which may cause pins and needles during this movement.

Exercise 30 Hamstrings – using a stool

Starting position and instructions
Stand in front of a waist-high stool and place your right foot on it. Keeping your right leg straight, lean forwards, moving from the hip while maintaining correct spinal alignment.

Variations
Hold on to an object or place your hand on a wall to increase the stability of the movement.

Points to note
Pulling your toes towards you and flexing your head and trunk will increase the stretch on the neural tissues and take the stretch away from the hamstring muscles.

Exercise 31 Hamstrings – using a bench

Starting position and instructions
Sit with your left leg straight along a bench, and your right leg flexed at the knee and pressed back into extension of the hip. Lean forwards, attempting to reach the foot of your left leg.

Variations
Releasing the full knee extension will increase the emphasis on the upper portion of the hamstrings.

Points to note
The pelvis should not tilt when extending the hip; no more than 15 degrees of extension is required.

Exercise 32 ITB – upper portion

Starting position and instructions

Lie on your back on a mat. Keep your right leg straight and flat on the mat. Bend your left leg to 90 degrees at the knee and hook your left calf over the top of your right leg. Press your pelvis down on the mat and use your right hand to press your left hip into adduction. Hold the stretched position for 30–60 seconds and then repeat the movement on the other side of the body.

Variations

Altering the amount of hip and knee flexion will vary the effect of the stretch.

Points to note

The ITB (ilio-tibial band) may be tight when the tensor fascia lata muscle that inserts into it is overworked. This can cause pain along the outside of the hip and thigh which this stretch can help to ease. The pain-relieving aspect of this movement can be enhanced by pressing into any painful spots (trigger points) along the outer edge of the hip while performing the stretch. Hold the pressure until the pain begins to subside.

Exercise 33 ITB – whole length

Starting position and instructions

Lie on your left side with your left leg slightly bent for support and your left arm above your head. Lift your right leg upwards and sideways (abduction) and press the left side of your body firmly into the mat. Allow the upper leg to lower down on to the mat (adduction).

Variations

Slightly flexing or extending the upper hip (moving it forwards or backwards, respectively) will alter the effect of this movement.

Points to note

The aim of this exercise is to adduct the top hip without allowing the pelvis to tilt sideways. This is achieved by flattening the side of the trunk against the mat and maintaining this position as the stretch is performed. If the pelvis is allowed to move, even slightly, the stretch will be ineffective. If your ITB is flexible, you may not notice this stretch achieving anything. Only when the ITB is tight do you feel the stretch over the outside of the hip. This exercise can also be performed with a partner holding your pelvis level.

Exercise 34 Deep calf and Achilles

Exercise 35 Toe flexion and extension

(a)   (b)

Starting position and instructions

Place a low stool or chair against a wall. Put your left foot in the centre of the chair and your right foot on the floor and slightly to the side of the chair and take up a lunge position. Keeping your foot flat, and your heel in contact with the chair seat, press your knee forwards over your toes.

Variations

Altering the angle of the foot away from the perpendicular will change the emphasis on the deep calf and Achilles.

Points to note

The heel must remain on the chair seat throughout the movement. Raising the heel takes the emphasis away from the deep calf and Achilles and throws it on to the foot itself. By bending the knee, the emphasis is taken away from the long superficial calf muscle (gastrocnemius) and placed on the shorter deep calf muscles (soleus and tibialis posterior).

Starting position and instructions

Stand with your feet bare and your hand against a wall for support. Point your foot (plantarflex) and press the ball of your foot into a mat (see (a) above), forcing your toes to bend upwards (extend). Hold the position for 10 seconds and then release. Pause, and then press the backs of your toes into the mat (see (b) above), encouraging your toes to bend downwards (flex).

Variations

If you find this stretch uncomfortable, press your toes on to a cushion or folded towel placed on the mat.

Points to note

Encourage this movement, but do not force it. Some individuals may have arthritic changes in their big toe joint (hallux rigidus), which will restrict the free movement of the joint and will require specialist physiotherapy.

Exercise 36 Plantar fascia

Exercise 37 Peronei muscles

Starting position and instructions

With your feet bare, stand in a supported lunge position with your hands against a wall. Gently press the ball of your back foot into a mat, pressing your knee downwards and forwards to encourage plantarflexion of your ankle.

Variations

You can alter the degree of either the knee or toe flexion (or both) to vary this stretch.

Points to note

The plantar fascia in the sole of the foot is tightened by a combination of toe flexion and ankle plantarflexion to wind the fascia around the ball of the foot as the arch of the foot is raised. Both actions combined are required, and either one performed on its own is less effective.

Starting position and instructions

Sit on a bench with your legs crossed, the ankle of your left leg over the knee of the right. Place your left hand on your left shin (medial malleolus) to stabilise the leg, and hook the fingers of your right hand around the outside of your left foot. Draw your foot inwards (inversion) and downwards (plantarflexion) with your right hand as you push against your left ankle with your left hand. Hold this position for 10–20 seconds and then reverse the exercise to stretch the right leg.

Variations

Altering the relative amounts of plantarflexion and inversion of the foot will change the emphasis of the stretch.

Points to note

To take the strain off your fingers, use your forearm and hand to pull your foot inwards.

Exercise 38 Lower back extension – lying

Starting position and instructions

Lie on the floor on your front and place your hands on the floor in the 'press-up' position. Push with your arms to arch your spine, keeping your hips firmly on the floor. Pause in the upper position and then lower. This movement stretches the rectus abdominis muscle and corrects any pressure imbalance in the lower back discs caused by prolonged sitting or lifting.

Variations

Pushing from your forearms until your elbows are locked at 90 degrees will limit the range of motion; pulling your arms towards your shoulders will increase the range of motion.

Points to note

This movement should be encouraged rather than forced, and repeated rhythmically to gain a pumping action on the discs of your lower spine. You should feel the stretch, but not pain, in the lower back. If you experience any pain, stop immediately.

Exercise 39 Thoracic spine rotation – lying

Starting position and instructions

Lie on the floor with your legs comfortably apart, and your arms out in a 'T' position. Stretch your right arm across your body, aiming to touch your left hand, and rotate your trunk to the left at the same time. This movement stretches the thoracic spine and the oblique abdominals and latissimus dorsi muscles of the upper side of the body.

Variations

Increasing the amount of abduction of your legs will increase the stability of the movement.

Points to note

Keeping your hips still will increase the emphasis of the stretch on your thoracic spine.

Exercise 40 Full spine rotation – standing

Starting position and instructions
Stand with your feet apart and arms out in a 'T' position. Rotate to the left, leading with your left arm, and then reverse the movement. This exercise stretches the oblique abdominals.

Variations
Lowering your arms and leading just with the shoulders reduces the overload.

Points to note
The leverage and momentum from your arms make it essential that the movement is performed in a slow and controlled fashion.

Exercise 41 Spinal rotation – lying: (a) normal (b) extreme movement range

(a)   (b)

Starting position and instructions
Lie on the floor with your left arm out at 90 degrees. Flex your left knee and rotate your trunk towards the right leg, bringing your left knee towards the floor. Place overpressure on the stretch by pressing your left knee to the floor using your right arm. The main emphasis of this stretch is on the oblique abdominals, but it also stretches the latissimus dorsi and anterior deltoid of the horizontal arm.

Variations
If you find the stretch too difficult, place a cushion on the floor and take your knee down on to the cushion. Alternatively, altering the degree of flexion at your hip and knee will alter the stress of the stretch.

Points to note
Because this action involves leverage, it should be performed in a slow and controlled manner. As the rotation occurs, the lower hip will tuck under the body. This is desirable, as it becomes the pivot point around which the body moves.

Exercise 42 Spinal rotation – two legs: (a) normal (b) extreme movement range

(a)

(b)

Starting position and instructions

Lie on the floor with your knees and hips flexed. Take your knees to the right side of your body and your arms out to the sides, maintaining the stretch. The main emphasis of this stretch is on the oblique abdominals, but it also stretches the latissimus dorsi and anterior deltoid of the upper arm.

Variations

Place a small cushion on the floor and lower your knees on to the cushion to reduce the range of motion if you find this exercise difficult.

Points to note

Due to the weight of your legs, they should be lowered slowly; dropping your legs is potentially dangerous for your spine.

Exercise 43 Spinal rotation – sitting (assisted)

Starting position and instructions

Sit on a stool or low bench, place your right arm behind the small of your back and grip the elbow of your left arm with your right hand. Twist to the right, leading the movement with the left hand. This exercise stretches the oblique abdominals.

Variations

If you are unable to grip your elbow, a looped towel may be used around the elbow instead.

Points to note

It is usual to have some degree of asymmetry, so rotation to the right and left sides may not be equal.

Exercise 44 Lateral flexion – standing

right   wrong

Exercise 45 Lateral flexion – with overpressure

Starting position and instructions

Stand with your feet apart. Laterally flex your spine, placing your right arm on your waist or thigh to support your bodyweight. Take your left arm above your head to increase the stretch. This movement stretches the latissimus dorsi and external oblique on the right side of the body.

Variations

Place both arms on the waist to reduce the overload. Stretching both hands overhead increases the overload on the spine, and changes the emphasis of the exercise from stretch to strength.

Points to note

Asymmetry of the lateral flexion of the spine is common, so movements may not be equal on both sides.

Starting position and instructions

Kneel on the floor and reach above your head with your left arm to lead a lateral flexion movement. Your right arm acts as a pivot by pressing the side of your ribcage. This exercise stretches the external oblique and the quadratus lumborum on the right side of the body.

Variations

Instead of taking your arm above your head, place both arms on your hips to reduce the overload on your spine.

Points to note

Asymmetry in this area is common, so movements may not be equal on both sides.

Exercise 46 Trunk lateral shift

Exercise 47 Trunk lateral shift – against a wall

Starting position and instructions

Stand with your arms out in a 'T' position. Lunge to the side with your left hand to shift the trunk. This exercise stretches the external oblique and quadratus lumborum on the left side of the body.

Variations

Performing the exercise with your back against a wall will ensure maximum alignment; performing in front of a mirror will often make the movement easier to control.

Points to note

The movement should come from your hips, with your shoulders remaining fairly static.

Starting position and instructions

Stand right-side-on to a wall with your right arm abducted to 90 degrees, your elbow bent and your forearm supported on the wall. Keep your shoulders still and press the right side of your pelvis and hips towards the wall.

Variations

If your posture type means that your spine leans more to one side than the other, perform the exercise only on that side. This is because the side flexor muscles on the side you lean towards will be shorter, and therefore require more stretching. For example, if your spine leans to the right, your right side flexor muscles will be tighter than those on the left. Pressing the pelvis to the right is actually equivalent to leaning over to the left (when the shoulders move to the left, the pelvis moves to the right), which stretches the right side of the body.

Points to note

There is very little movement in this exercise, so the action is one of a subtle press or squeeze rather than a noticeable muscle stretch.

Exercise 48 Skull rock

Exercise 49 Cervical spine flexion – with overpressure

Starting position and instructions

Lie on your back on a mat. Relax your shoulders and keep the back of your head on the mat throughout the movement. Gently draw your chin in, as though trying to press your chin into the top of your breastbone.

Variations

This exercise can also be performed while standing, with your head and shoulders resting against a wall. Also, to increase the effect of the stretch you can assist the movement by placing overpressure on your chin with your hands. This movement emphasises the stretch on the upper part of the cervical spine.

Points to note

As you perform this action, the back of the skull should move in a line up and down the mat by about 10 cm. If you find that your head does not rest on the mat easily, place one or two thin books underneath your head until the resting position suits your posture.

Starting position and instructions

Sit on a gym bench, interlace your fingers and place your hands behind your head. Bend your neck to look downwards towards your chest, then place overpressure on this movement by pulling gently on the back of your head with your hands. Maintain the stretched position for 10 seconds and then repeat. Perform 3 repetitions only.

Variations

You can also stretch the upper part of the thoracic spine by allowing the shoulders to round slightly. To restrict the movement to the upper cervical spine, try to draw the chin into the lower part of the throat instead of looking down at the chest.

Points to note

As the neck is a delicate structure, the overpressure used in this stretch must be small and controlled. Use very light pressure from the hands to guide the neck, rather than forcing the movement. Do not perform high repetitions of this movement; 3 is the maximum required.

Exercise 50 Cervical rotation – with overpressure

Starting position and instructions

Sit on a gym bench with your spine correctly aligned. Turn your head to the right and assist the movement by gently pressing on to the angle of your jaw with your left hand. Aim to bring your chin over the point of your shoulder.

Variations

The rotation movement can also be combined with either flexion (look down towards the floor) or extension (look up at the ceiling).

Points to note

As you turn your head, be careful not to turn your trunk as well by twisting the shoulders, as this will release some of the stretch. The neck should move relative to the shoulders, not with them.

Exercise 51 Jaw joint

Starting position and instructions

Sit in front of a mirror. Open your mouth and place one bent finger between your teeth. Maintain this stretch for 10–20 seconds and then remove the finger and close your mouth. Repeat the stretch, this time using two fingers and, eventually (after many weeks), using three.

Variations

If your jaw is so tight that you are unable to even get one finger between your teeth, use a thinner object such as a toothbrush handle at first.

Points to note

The jaw joint (tempero mandibular joint or TMJ) is controlled by the powerful biting muscles. In individuals who have a tendency to grind their teeth at night, these muscles become short and tight. To stretch them effectively may take weeks, gradually increasing the movement by a few millimetres each day. As the stretch is placed on the joint, try to relax the jaw and allow the stretch to take effect. Avoid the temptation to actually 'bite' the finger and tense the jaw muscles.

Exercise 52 Rhomboids and thoracic spine

Starting position and instructions

Sitting on a bench, cross your arms across your chest placing each of your hands on its opposite shoulder, and flex your trunk at the thoracic spine.

Variations

Combine the flexion movement with rotation and/or lateral flexion to change the emphasis on the thoracic spine. If you feel pain between your shoulder blades that is relieved by this movement, the pain is often caused by spasms within the rhomboid muscles. Pain relief can be enhanced by having someone gently press their thumbs into the muscles between the spine and the inner (medial) edge of the scapula while in the stretched position.

Points to note

This exercise should be used with caution, as this area of the spine is quite often too flexible (hyperflexible).

Exercise 53 Anterior chest and shoulders

Starting position and instructions

Stand in front of a doorway or in the corner of a room with your shoulders and elbows flexed to 90 degrees. Lean forwards, pressing your chest through the space in front of you and forcing your arms back into extension.

Variations

Increasing and reducing the height of the arms will vary the focus of the stretch.

Points to note

Because the full bodyweight is being supported, heavy individuals and those with poor shoulder flexibility should take up a lunge position, moving some of the bodyweight on to the front foot.

Exercise 54 Pectoralis – minor muscle

Starting position and instructions

Lie on your back on a mat. Tuck your left hand beneath the outside of your left hip and place a small ball such as a squash ball between the back of your left shoulder and the mat. The squash ball should be level with the ball of the joint rather than your shoulder blade. Firmly press your shoulder back into the mat, trying to compress the squash ball. Hold the stretched position for 20–30 seconds and then release.

Variations

Pressing on to a squash ball is an active stretch and requires the strength of your shoulder retractor muscles to be greater than the tightness of your shoulder protractor muscles. However, if your shoulder is very tight, it may be better to perform the exercise passively by asking your training partner to press your shoulder down using the flat of their hand.

Points to note

As you perform the action, try not to rotate the trunk and ribcage to the side as this will release the stretching force. Instead, keep the ribcage relatively fixed as the shoulder is stretched.

Exercise 55 Upper trapezius

Starting position and instructions

Sit on a stool or bench and grip the stool top with your right hand. Laterally flex your neck to the left allowing your right shoulder to elevate. Fix your neck in position with your left hand, and actively depress your right shoulder to overload the stretch.

Variations

Flex and extend your head to change the emphasis of the stretch.

Points to note

The power from the stretch must be from pulling the shoulder downwards rather than pulling on the neck, since the neck is the more delicate of the two structures.

Exercise 56 Shoulder adductors and extensors

Starting position and instructions
Grip a high point and straighten your arms. Keeping your hands fixed, bend your knees and lower your body down and back, feeling the stretch beneath your arms. This movement stretches the latissimus dorsi and the triceps muscles.

Variations
Altering the position of the hands will change the exact point of the stretch.

Points to note
Gripping a higher point will increase the range of motion, but reduce the bodyweight placed on the stretch. Gripping a lower point will encourage you to lean back and take more weight through your shoulders.

Exercise 57 Shoulder rotation – lying

Starting position and instructions
Lie on your back on a mat with your arms abducted and elbows flexed to 90 degrees. Allow your forearms to fall back into the horizontal position, rotating the shoulders. This position stretches the shoulder rotators.

Variations
Alter the angle of abduction at the shoulder to vary the exact site of the stretch.

Points to note
With the use of weights, this exercise is ideal for contract–relax techniques.

Exercise 58 Shoulder rotation – weight overload

Starting position and instructions

Lie on the floor and grip a weight bag in your left hand. Place your upper arm close to your body and flex your elbow to 90 degrees. Allow the weight of the bag to force your shoulder into external rotation. This position stretches the shoulder rotators.

Variations

Increasing and reducing the weight will change the intensity of the stretch.

Points to note

Since a weight is used, this exercise is ideal for contract–relax techniques. Try to ensure that the shoulder does not move forwards as the stretch is placed on the shoulder. Keep the back of the shoulder in contact with the mat throughout the movement.

Exercise 59 Forearm pronation and wrist flexion

Starting position and instructions

Stand with your arms by your sides. Pronate your right forearm and flex your right wrist. Grip your right wrist with your left hand and press your right wrist into further flexion.

Variations

This exercise can be combined with radial or ulnar deviation to maximally stress your extensor carpi radialis longus muscle.

Points to note

For cases of tennis elbow, combining the wrist flexion and ulnar deviation will maximally stress your extensor carpi radialis longus muscle.

Exercise 60 Wrist extensors – with self overpressure

Starting position and instructions
Straighten your right arm and flex your right wrist. Grip your right hand with your left, placing your left thumb into the crease of your right wrist. Using your left thumb as a pivot, pull your right wrist into full flexion.

Variations
Altering the position of the thumb will localise the stretch.

Points to note
Because of the leverage involved, the stretch must be slow and controlled.

Exercise 61 Wrist extensors – against a wall

Starting position and instructions
Stand facing a wall, place the back of your right hand flat on the wall with your fingers vertical and straighten your arm. Use your left hand to lock your right elbow and maintain the locked position throughout the movement. Lean forwards towards the wall, pressing your wrist into further flexion.

Variations
Placing your hand higher up the wall will increase the range of motion.

Points to note
Where an ache is felt close to the elbow, the muscle is being stretched, but where the sensation is over the wrist, the wrist extensor tendons and tissue are being stretched.

Exercise 62 Wrist flexors

Exercise 63 Wrist abduction and adduction

Starting position and instructions

Straighten your right arm and, with your left hand, take hold of the palm of your right hand below the knuckles and pull your right hand back in to extension. Hold the stretch for 10 seconds and then repeat.

Variations

Placing the thumb of the left hand in the crease at the back of the right hand will localise the stretch to the area of the wrist.

Points to note

There are seven small carpal bones within the wrist; this exercise will stretch all of the wrist, but will not isolate the stretch to a single bone. If a single joint is stiff, manual therapy from a physiotherapist will be required.

Starting position and instructions

Place your right forearm on a low table with your hand flat and fingers spread. Place your left hand over your right to prevent your hand from sliding on the tabletop. Glide your forearm from side to side, encouraging abduction and adduction at the wrist.

Variations

Both abduction and adduction can be combined with a slight amount of flexion or extension to vary the stretch.

Points to note

There is always more adduction (movement towards the little finger) than abduction (movement towards the thumb) available at the wrist.

Exercise 64 Finger flexors

Starting position and instructions
Grip one finger of your right hand. Place the forefinger of your left hand underneath the first finger. Pull the finger back into extension. Repeat on all fingers.

Variations
Combining extension with abduction and adduction will vary the site of the stretch.

Points to note
Because of the leverage involved, the stretch must be slow and controlled.

Exercise 65 Finger flexors and palm of the hand

Starting position and instructions
Place the tips of your fingers and thumbs together. Press your hands closer together to force your fingers and thumbs into extension. Hold the stretch for 10 seconds and then repeat.

Variations
Because the tissues being stretched are superficial, heat will increase the range of motion. The exercise can therefore be performed with the hands submerged in warm water.

Points to note
Individuals who have extremely lax finger joints may find that their distal interphalangeal joint hyperextends. If this is the case, they should start with the fingers flexed first and then stretch to the mid-position only.

Exercise 66 Finger adductors

Starting position and instructions

Place your right hand on a flat surface and place the thumb and index finger of your left hand between two of the right. Force the right-hand fingers apart.

Variations

A small golf ball can be used between your fingers instead of the thumb and finger of your other hand. Pressing the golf ball closer to the web of your hand increases the range of motion obtained with the stretch.

Points to note

Because of the leverage involved, the stretch must be slow and controlled. In individuals where the distal interphalangeal joints are hypermobile, the stretch can be placed closer to the finger web.

ADVANCED STRETCHES

9

Exercise 67 Hip flexors and extensors – modified lunge

Starting position and instructions
Start with your feet shoulder width apart. Step forwards with your left leg and lower your body towards the ground, supporting your weight with your hands. Keep your left foot flat and your knee and foot in line.

Variations
Placing the hands inside the knee will increase the available range of motion.

Points to note
Because full bodyweight is being used, the exercise must be performed slowly.

Exercise 68 Hip flexors and extensors – extended range

Exercise 69 Hip adductors – standing

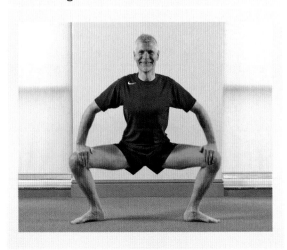

Starting position and instructions

Start with your feet shoulder width apart. Step forwards with your left leg and lower your body towards the ground, supporting your weight with your hands. Turn your left knee outwards and your left foot inwards to bring the left thigh down on to the ground, with the left heel on the inside of your groin. At the same time, slide your right leg backwards to bring it down on to the mat.

Variations

Bending your right knee will increase the stretch on the rectus femoris of your right leg. Instead of turning your left knee out and bringing your heel to the inside of the groin, you can simply sit on the heel of your left leg. This reduces the stretch on the gluteal muscles of the left leg, but also takes away any rotation strain on the knee.

Points to note

This is an extreme stretch and as such should only be practised after the basic stretch for the hip flexors and extensors (*see* exercise 67, page 139) has been mastered. The exercise should be performed slowly, keeping control of the bodyweight at all times by lowering the body with the hands.

Starting position and instructions

Stand with your feet wide apart and your toes pointing out. Squat down until your thighs are at 90 degrees to your calves, placing your hands on your knees. Press with your hands to force your knees into further abduction.

Variations

Hold on to your ankles and press your knees apart with your elbows.

Points to note

This movement is quite unstable, so some individuals may find it easier to support their weight on a stool.

Exercise 70 Hip adductors and rotators

Points to note
This exercise causes extreme 'turn out' (hip lateral rotation) and so is popular with ballet students. However, it must be used with caution as the leverage forces are quite high. In children, any movement that forces the hip can be dangerous and if pain occurs in the hip joint rather than in the muscles, the movement must be stopped immediately. In seniors, this movement should not be attempted if you have had a hip joint replacement or hip surgery of any type.

Starting position and instructions
Lie on your front in the 'frog' position: your hips should be flexed, abducted and laterally rotated (turned out). Your knees should be bent to 90 degrees and your feet should be touching. From this position, try to straighten your legs and touch the floor with your toes, without allowing the front of your hips to leave the mat.

Variations
Rather than beginning with your hips on the mat and attempting to touch the mat with your toes, you can begin with your toes on the mat (in which case your hips will lift off the mat) and attempt to lower your hips down. As the hips are heavier than the shins, this action gives greater overpressure.

Exercise 71 Hip adductors – with trunk lateral flexion

Starting position and instructions

Place your left foot on a waist-high object with your toes pointing forwards and laterally flex your trunk to the left.

Variations

Altering the height of the object will vary the stretch. Taking the right arm overhead will increase the stretch.

Points to note

Because you are standing on one leg, this exercise is unstable; if you need to, hold on to an object throughout the movement. The upper arm must reach towards the foot, not press downwards on the outside of the knee. Because of the stress placed on the knee, this exercise is unsuitable if you have had a knee ligament injury.

Exercise 72 Gluteals

Starting position and instructions

Lie on your back on the floor, flex your left hip and rotate it. Draw your right knee up, pressing your knee on to your left foot. Reach around your right knee and pull your knee towards your shoulder, forcing your left hip into external rotation.

Variations

Altering the angle of hip motion of your left leg will change the emphasis of the stretch.

Points to note

This exercise also places stress on the pelvis, so it is inappropriate after pregnancy. If you are unable to flex your hip high enough to grip around your thigh, loop a towel around your thigh and grip that instead.

Exercise 73 Gluteals - increased range

Starting position and instructions
Lie on the floor on your back. Bend your right hip and knee and link your right arm around your shin, taking your forearm under the knee and to the outside of your shin. Hold your right foot in your interlocked hands. Keeping your knee at 90-degree flexion, draw your foot in towards your face.

Variations
Take your foot higher (over your head) or lower (over your chest) to vary the stretch intensity.

Points to note
When you lie down, your head may not rest on the floor comfortably. If this is the case, do not allow it to drop back into extension but place a folded towel or foam block beneath your head for support and alignment.

Exercise 74 Hamstrings and hip adductors - lying

Starting position and instructions
Lie on your back on the floor with both legs straight. Take your right leg into flexion and then out into abduction, aiming to rest it on the floor. Keep both shoulders and hips on the floor.

Variations
Place a small cushion or block under your leg to limit the full movement.

Points to note
The subject must be strong to lower the leg under control, and under no circumstances should the leg be dropped rapidly towards the floor.

Exercise 75 Hamstrings and hip adductors – splits position with stool support

Starting position and instructions
Stand with your feet apart and then slide them out to form a splits position. Flex your trunk at the hip and place your forearms on a stool or two to three yoga blocks to support your bodyweight.

Variations
Place your feet on a shiny piece of paper (on a carpet surface) or cloth (on a wooden floor) to allow your feet to slide more easily. If you are very flexible, you may be able to dispense with the stool and place your forearms flat on the floor. However, if you do this make sure that you maintain your spinal alignment; do not perform extreme spinal flexion simply to put your arms on the floor. It is better to use a stool and maintain spinal alignment. The effect on hip flexibility is the same in both cases.

Points to note
Your pelvis should remain above your hips throughout the movement and your bodyweight must be taken on your forearms to reduce the stress on your knees. This exercise is unsuitable if you have had a knee ligament injury, as it stresses the inner (medial) ligament of the knee.

Exercise 76 Hamstrings and hip adductors – splits position to head

Starting position and instructions
This is a progression to exercise 75 and should only be performed when that exercise can be practised easily. Stand with your feet apart, then slide them out to form a maximal splits position. Take your bodyweight back on to your heels and flex your trunk at the hip, bending forwards to place your head on the ground.

Variations
Initially, you may find this exercise easier if you sit on a low stool or some stacked yoga blocks.

Points to note
It is essential to take your bodyweight backwards on to your heels in this movement. As you place your head on to the ground, at least two-thirds of your bodyweight should be supported by your legs and one-third by your head, purely for balance. This is an extreme movement that is popular with dancers, gymnasts and martial artists. It requires excellent muscle strength and muscle control and should not be attempted by people with poor fitness levels. Even when performed by optimally fit individuals, this stretch places considerable strain on the inner (medial) ligament of the knee. A single repetition only should be performed and held for 10–30 seconds maximum.

Exercise 77 Spinal rotation – using leg leverage

Exercise 78 Full spine rotation – with overpressure

Starting position and instructions

Lie on your front with your head supported by your crossed arms. Take your right leg up and across your body to touch the floor on your left, twisting your trunk and flexing your knee as the movement progresses. This exercise stretches the oblique abdominals.

Variations

Altering the degree of flexion at your knee and the extension of your hip will change the emphasis of the stretch.

Points to note

Due to the weight of your leg, it should be lowered under control rather than forcing your spine into extension and rotation.

Starting position and instructions

Stand with your feet slightly apart. Cross your right foot over your left to rotate your pelvis and hips to the left. Twist your trunk to the right, bringing your left arm in front of you and your right arm behind you. Grip the inside of your left elbow with your right hand and use your left arm to pull your right side into further rotation.

Variations

If lack of shoulder flexibility limits your ability to grip your elbow, fold a towel around your left elbow to grip instead.

Points to note

The overpressure that this exercise can generate is quite high. Be careful therefore to keep the action slow and controlled throughout, avoiding the tendency to 'bounce' into the movement.

Exercise 79 Lateral flexion and rotation

Starting position and instructions
Stand with your feet wide apart and turn your right foot out (lateral rotation of the hip). Reach down towards your right shin or ankle with your right arm and point your left arm towards the ceiling to offer counterbalance. This exercise stretches the oblique abdominals and the quadratus lumborum.

Variations
Allow your upper arm to rest on your body to alter the stress.

Points to note
Your bodyweight must be taken through your arm on to your shin or ankle throughout the movement to reduce the leverage (stress) on your spine. If you have a history of lower back pain, you should only attempt this exercise under the supervision of a qualified instructor.

Exercise 80 Lower back extension – standing

Starting position and instructions
Stand with your feet hip width apart and your hands at the top of your buttocks. Extend your spine by pressing your hips forwards, pushing with your hands and at the same time looking upwards. Perform the exercise (lumbar extension) slowly and rhythmically, but do not hold it in the upward position as this is quite stressful on the lower back.

Variations
This action can be combined with rotation and/or lateral flexion if the combined movement seems to be stiffer than the pure movement.

Points to note
When the action is stiff and painful, perform it for 3–5 repetitions only. If the pain subsides, the exercise can be continued; if the pain does not subside, rest and then repeat the action; if the pain increases, stop immediately. If you do not press the hips forwards, the extension action becomes a simple 'lean back'. Because of the effect of the gravity line of the body, this places more compression on the lumbar spine than performing the action by moving the hips forwards.

Exercise 81 Anterior chest and shoulders

Starting position and instructions
Standing side-on to a wall, place your right hand on the wall at shoulder height. Keeping your right arm straight, turn your feet to the left and rotate your body to the left, feeling the stretch across the front of your right shoulder. This movement stretches the anterior deltoid, pectoral and biceps muscles.

Variations
Altering the height of the hand on the wall will vary the site of the stretch.

Points to note
Because of the momentum involved in this exercise, the trunk twist must be slow and controlled at all times.

Exercise 82 Shoulder flexors

Starting position and instructions
Keeping your arms straight, extend them behind you and place the backs of your hands on a high table or windowsill. Maintaining correct body alignment, bend your knees to lower your body, pressing your shoulders into further extension. This movement stretches the anterior deltoid, pectoral and biceps muscles.

Variations
Putting your hands closer together or further apart changes the muscle emphasis of the exercise.

Points to note
In cases of shoulder dislocation, this exercise should not be used: as the arm is forced back into extension, the ball of the shoulder (head of the humerus) moves forwards in the joint, stressing the anterior structures.

Exercise 83 Forearm flexors

Exercise 84 Thumb flexors and abductors

Starting position and instructions

Place your right hand flat against a wall with your fingers pointing to the floor and your right arm straight. Hold your right elbow locked using your left hand. Lean your bodyweight forwards, pressing the heel of your right hand into the wall.

Variations

Placing your hand higher up the wall will increase the stretch.

Points to note

Releasing the elbow even very slightly will make the stretch less effective.

Starting position and instructions

Place your right hand palm up with your thumb extended. With your left hand, grip your right thumb from beneath and pull your thumb into extension and abduction.

Variations

Altering the exact position of the thumb will vary the site of the stretch.

Points to note

Because of the leverage involved in this stretch, the force applied should be slow and continuous rather than sudden.

PARTNER STRETCHES

10

The stretches described in this book so far have only been applied by the user. However, stretches can also be applied by a second person, be it a training partner, personal trainer, or clinical therapist.

Partner stretches are useful because they enable the user to relax while your partner supplies the force for the stretch. Furthermore because a second person is observing movement from outside the moving body, alignment can be improved. In addition, working with a partner can boost motivation.

However, there is one thing you should be careful of with partner stretches. When you perform a stretch by yourself, the sensation you feel in the muscles is used to limit the force that you apply. In short, if it hurts, you stop. With partner stretches, however, your partner cannot feel your pain, so you must keep him or her informed throughout the stretch about exactly how the exercise feels.

Key point:

Partner stretches can (i) ensure better body alignment, (ii) enable the user to relax as they are not producing muscle force, and (iii) motivate the user to increase the stretch intensity.

TISSUE RESISTANCE AT END RANGE

A physiotherapist or experienced personal trainer will be able to feel tissue tension – that is the feel of the tissue as it is stretched. When you stretch and get to the end of your movement, the feeling of the tissues is important, and in clinical terms is called movement end feel (table 10.1).

End feel is the sensation that the therapist feels through their hands when the movement of the joint stops at the end of a stretching action. A *hard* end feel indicates that bone is limiting movement,

Table 10.1	Joint end feel
Movement range	**End feel**
NORMAL (full range)	
• Hard • Soft • Elastic	• Bone on bone • Flesh (soft tissue) against flesh • Tissues on stretch
ABNORMAL (range is limited)	
• Hard • Springy • Empty	• Complete block, often accompanied by joint grating (crepitus) on movement • Movement stops prematurely as though something is caught in a joint • Movement halted prematurely by client's action alone

and a typical example would be elbow extension as the arm locks out straight. Clearly, bone cannot be stretched, so when the tissue tension feel is hard, a personal trainer will ease off as they know that no further stretch is possible. A *soft* end feel indicates that soft tissues such as muscle, fat and skin are pressing against each other to limit movement, the typical example being elbow flexion. Clearly movement range will be more limited in an obese individual as there is more soft tissue between the two limbs. This is a consideration for joint nutrition, because with day-to-day activities movement range will be reduced in an obese person and so joint nutrition will be reduced.

Finally, an *elastic* end feel occurs when tissues are stretched and limit the movement range. A typical example of an elastic end feel is a straight leg raise where the hamstrings are stretched. As the stretch continues, the elasticity also continues but is not as strong, a little like the difference between stretching a thick elastic band and then stretching a thinner one. How quickly the end feel changes is also important because it shows us how someone will respond to stretching. In clinical terms we can talk about the onset of resistance (delineated on a client's notes as 'R1'), and the final point at which no further movement is possible (written on the notes as 'R2'). R1 is sometimes referred to as the physiological end range, in other words the range at which the body tissues tense up to stiffen the movement and protect a body part. This occurs both through muscle tightening (increased tone) and wind up of connective tissue. R2 represents anatomical end range – the final degree of movement which is possible. So for example if you stretch a person's joint you will get to R1, but if they were put under an anaesthetic so all of their muscles were relaxed, and you warmed all of the tissues to make them pliable, you could go further and eventually reach R2.

These three types of end feel can all be viewed as normal in each case, but represent different limitations to motion range. Abnormal end feels include a *springy* sensation where something is trapped in a joint and an *empty* end feel where muscles go into spasm to block the final degrees of movement and protect the joint. This becomes more obvious when one side of the body has markedly less movement than the other and the action is painful. When an abnormal end feel is felt by your training partner or personal trainer during partner stretching, you should be referred to a physiotherapist for further examination.

There are both advantages and disadvantages of partner work. On the plus side, motivation is better, but on the minus side, the exercise is less controlled because two people are involved. Therefore, when practising partner stretches a stable starting position must be chosen to avoid either person falling and violently increasing the stretch. The two partners act as one unit, so their combined mass has a single base of support and a single line of gravity (*see* pages 11–12), with the base of support being larger than it would be for a single person. The person applying the stretch must move into a comfortable position that they can easily maintain, rather than moving into an awkward position that places them off balance so that they have to continuously readjust their position.

If partner activities are used in a group exercise situation, they must be practised under the supervision of an experienced and skilled instructor. Close supervision of individuals in the group is essential, especially when dealing with young or inexperienced people. When teaching partner work to adolescents, they should be matched for body size and degree of flexibility.

Key point:

An abnormal end feel of a joint during partner stretching is a reason for referral to a registered physiotherapist.

Exercise 85 Hip flexors – supine lying

Starting position and instructions

Lie on the floor with your left hip and knee flexed. Your partner half kneels at your left hip. With their left hand they hold your right leg on the floor, and with their right hand they press your left leg into further hip flexion. This movement stretches the rectus femoris and iliopsoas of the lower leg, and the gluteals of the upper leg.

Variations

For those who experience pain in their knee, the partner's hand should be positioned on the underside of the knee. If you are performing this action on a bench or treatment couch, the leg should be held close to your body for control. Your hands are placed on the back of your client's thigh, below the knee to avoid pressing into the delicate structures at the back of the knee (popliteal fossa).

Points to note

Most individuals are asymmetrical, so one leg may appear less flexible than the other.

Exercise 86 Hip distraction – lying

Starting position and instructions

Begin with your partner/client lying on a gym bench or treatment couch. Hold their left leg securely by cradling it in the crook of your left arm. Lock the position by placing your right hand on top of their leg and gripping your right arm with your left hand (4-lock position). Their leg should be in a loose-pack position (*see* chapter 2) of slight hip flexion, abduction, and external rotation. Gradually lean backwards to impart a distraction force on their leg. Hold the position for 30 seconds and then release.

Variations

Perform an oscillation action (longitudinal joint mobilisation) by gently distracting and then releasing your partner's leg in a rhythmic fashion for 20–30 repetitions.

Points to note

Very little force (2–5 lb) is required for this action. The aim is to allow your partner's muscles to relax completely as you apply the distraction force targeted at the joint structures. This action should not be used on an individual who has had a hip replacement or resurfacing operation, unless applied by a registered physiotherapist.

Exercise 87 Mobilisation with movement – using a belt

Starting position and instructions

Begin with your partner/client lying on their back on a gym couch with their left leg bent (flexed). Stand to their left side and hook a wide belt (seatbelt or yoga strap) around the top of their thigh, and then around your hips. Lean backwards on the belt to apply an outward (lateral) distraction force to the hip joint. Grasp their left thigh (femur) and press their knee towards their chest (hip flexion). Pause in the full range position for 5–10 seconds and then lower under control, releasing the distraction force applied through the belt.

Variations

Perform a rhythmic oscillation by pressing the hip into flexion and then releasing 5–10 times.

Key point:

Partner stretches introduce variety to training and are good for motivation. The danger of overstretching is ever present, however, so communication between partners is essential.

Points to note

When the hip is stiff or has been painful, it may move out of alignment with the ball, catching (impinging) on to the edge of the socket. The aim of this stretch is to keep the ball within the centre of the socket and prevent impingement. Very little force is required, and the amount can be judged by the effect. If the hip is painful at the point of maximum flexion, enough force is applied to reduce the pain. If pain increases, or does not reduce, the technique is not suitable for your partner's hip condition.

Exercise 88 Hip adductors – stride sitting

Exercise 89 Hip adductors – lying on bench

Starting position and instructions

Sit on the floor with your hips abducted. Your partner sits in front of you and places their feet on your inner shins. Link arms, and your partner presses your legs apart while pulling your trunk forwards. Hinge at the hips, keeping your spine aligned throughout the action.

Variations

Instead of pulling arm to arm, your partner can place a towel around your waist and pull your trunk forwards by pulling on the towel. This reduces the leverage on the spine.

Points to note

There must be equal pressure between pressing with the feet and pulling on the trunk to increase flexibility. The aim of the trunk pull is simply to encourage pelvic tilt, moving the buttocks (ischial tuberosity) backwards in relation to the knee. When trunk flexion occurs, the stretch has moved from the adductors to the trunk tissues.

Starting position and instructions

Begin with your partner lying on a gym bench or treatment couch. Stand to their left side and hold their left leg securely. Loop your right arm beneath their thigh and use your left arm to stabilise their pelvis. Draw their left leg outwards in a scissor action (hip abduction), holding the full range position for 10–20 seconds.

Variations

Perform a PNF stretch by having your partner draw their legs together (adduction) as you provide a resistance to match their force (isometric contraction). When they release the muscle contraction, pause for 5 seconds and then apply the stretch.

Points to note

As the hip moves into abduction there is a tendency for the leg to twist outwards (external rotation). If allowed, this will take some stretch from the adductors and place it on to the hamstring muscles.

153

Exercise 90 Hip adductors –sitting back to back

Points to note

As you are taking the weight of your partner's trunk on your own, there is a tendency for you to flex your spine excessively if your hips are very tight. If this occurs, the exercise is not suitable for you. Some bending (flexion) of the spine may occur, which should be balanced by straightening your spine (extension) as you stretch over your partner.

Starting position and instructions

Sit on the floor with your legs as far apart as possible. Your partner sits in the same position with their back to you. Sit close together with your tailbones touching. Lean forwards and place your hands on the ground, trying to bend from your waist only. At the same time, your partner reaches overhead with both arms and leans back on to you, extending their spine as you flex forwards. Hold the stretch position for 20–30 seconds and then reverse, reaching overhead and arching your back over your partner.

Variations

If you find that your back is bending too much, place three to four yoga blocks in front of you and lean your elbows on the blocks rather than placing your hands on the floor. Try to emphasise the movement of the hips by performing a forward (anterior) tilt of your pelvis and maintaining the hollow in the small of your back.

Exercise 91 Hip adductors and trunk side flexors – sitting back to back

Starting position and instructions

Sit back to back with your partner and abduct your hips into a stretched stride position. Link hands and lean to the right, bending your right arm and placing your forearm on the ground, pulling your partner to their left. Maintain this side-leaning position and reach your left arm overhead and to the right side, pulling your partner's right arm to the left as you do so. Maintain the position for 20–30 seconds and then reverse the movement, stretching to your left side.

Variations

Rather than holding hands with your partner, you can hold a stick or broom handle between you in an overhead grip. As you lean to the side, however, you will not be able to take your weight through your forearms, so be careful not to stretch too far.

Points to note

By gripping each other's hands, you avoid the tendency to bend forwards. However, you must make sure first, that you are both the same size so that your arm length matches, and second that one person does not pull excessively as you bend to the side.

Exercise 92 Hip abductors – side lying (Ober position)

Starting position and instructions

Lie on a bench or the floor on your left-hand side; your partner kneels behind you at waist level. Your partner abducts and extends your right leg with their right arm while fixing your pelvis with their left arm. Keeping the pelvis stable (avoiding any side tilt) and pressing your right leg down into adduction stretches the abductors.

Variations

Flexing the leg will emphasise the posterior portion of the gluteus medius.

Points to note

Allowing even a small amount of pelvic movement will completely release the stretch in this exercise. You will only feel the stretch if you have tightness in the hip abductors of the upper leg.

Exercise 93 Hip rotation – lying

Starting position and instructions

Lie on the floor on your back with your partner kneeling at your right-hand side by your waist. Your partner flexes your right knee and hip and presses it inwards and outwards, encouraging rotation at the hip. This movement stretches the medial and lateral rotators of the hip.

Variations

Altering the angle of hip flexion will vary the stress on the hip rotators.

Points to note

This exercise places stress on the pelvic joints, so it must be used with caution following pregnancy.

Exercise 94 Hamstrings – lying

Starting position and instructions

Lie on the floor with your legs straight. Your partner half kneels at your right hip and lifts your right leg, placing their hand over your knee to keep the leg straight. Your leg rests on your partner's shoulder and they lunge forwards, pressing your leg into further flexion at the hip.

Variations

Place a small pad on your partner's shoulder and a small rolled towel under your back to make the position more comfortable.

Points to note

This exercise is most effective when used with PNF techniques. When locking the leg out straight, make sure that the pressure is not placed directly over the kneecap. Cup your hand and place it around, but not directly on top of, your partner's knee.

Exercise 95 Hamstrings – standing (wall support)

Starting position and instructions
Stand with your back to a wall; your partner stands facing you in a lunge stance, knees slightly bent. Place your right leg on your partner's left shoulder, keeping your leg straight. Your partner gradually straightens their legs, pressing your right leg into further flexion.

Variations
If you are extremely flexible, your partner can place their hands together and hold your foot as they press your hip into further flexion above their shoulder. If you are less flexible, your partner can cup their hands around your leg and lift it to the level of their waist.

Points to note
Stability is important, so if you find you are unstable during this exercise, hold on to the wall.

Exercise 96 Gastrocnemius – lying

Starting position and instructions
Lie on the floor with partner half kneeling at your shins. Your partner places a folded towel beneath your left calf and cups their hand around your left heel. Get your partner to lunge forwards, pressing their forearm against your foot to push your foot into dorsiflexion (toes upwards).

Variations
Placing the folded towel beneath your knee, flex the knee throwing the stress from the long calf muscle (gastrocnemius) to the short calf muscle (soleus).

Points to note
The calf and Achilles are very powerful and often very tight. It is essential that your partner places the stretch on using their bodyweight rather than simply their hands. Using only the hands places considerable stress on the hand and finger joints.

Exercise 97 Flat back hamstring stretch – the 'table top'

Starting position and instructions

Stand facing your partner about half a body length apart with your feet hip width apart and your legs straight. Your partner should have their feet twice hip width apart and their knees slightly bent (soft). Hold hands with your partner and, keeping your trunk very straight, bend forwards at the hips and reach your arms out to rest at the level of your partner's hips. Your partner takes the weight of your upper body as you do so.

Variations

You can also perform this exercise by both leaning forwards. In this case, begin by standing a full body length apart and lean forwards slowly until you are able to hold hands. At the end of the movement, your upper bodies and arms should be completely flat and in line.

Points to note

The aim of this movement is to place the stretch on the hamstrings by tilting the pelvis forwards and keeping the spine straight or even slightly hollow in the lumbar spine (lumbar lordosis maintained). To facilitate this, pull your abdomen in and slightly brace your shoulders while pressing your chest outwards (thoracic extension). With the first movement, some of your bodyweight is taken by your partner. In the variation, you both support your own full weight and use each other purely for balance, therefore emphasising strength as well as stretch.

Exercise 98 Sit and reach – back to back

Exercise 99 Lower back flexion – sitting

Starting position and instructions

Sit on the floor back-to-back with your partner with your tailbones touching and your legs out straight. Lean forwards towards your toes, supporting your bodyweight by resting your forearms on your thighs or wherever is comfortable. At the same time, your partner reaches overhead with both arms and leans back on to you. Allow the overpressure of your partner's weight to press you further forwards, keeping your back as straight as possible.

Variations

To place less overload on the stretch, your partner can keep their arms by their sides rather than reaching overhead.

Points to note

This stretch relies on you both having approximately the same upper body length. If one of you is shorter, they can sit on one or two yoga blocks to bring your shoulders up to the same height. Also, if one person is heavier than the other, they will apply greater pressure simply through their bodyweight. Make sure, therefore, that you are weight-matched with your partner.

Starting position and instructions

Sit on a mat with your knees loosely bent and wider than hip width apart. Your partner kneels behind you. Bend forwards from the hips, placing a hand on the floor for support. At the end of the movement, your partner places overload on your lower back to increase the stretch.

Variations

Straightening the legs slightly throws extra stress on the hamstring muscles. Sitting with a folded towel or yoga block under your sitting bones (ischial tuberosities) tilts your pelvis forwards and assists alignment.

Points to note

The aim of this movement is to tilt the pelvis forwards with minimal spinal flexion. Overpressure must be placed on the lumbar spine and not between the shoulder blades. If your partner presses too high up, the tendency is to increase flexion of the thoracic spine rather than increasing the forward pelvic tilt.

Exercise 100 Rectus femoris stretch – lying

Starting position and instructions

Begin with your partner/client lying on a gym bench or treatment couch on their right side. Bend their left knee and support it with your left arm beneath their leg. Grip their thigh in your hand and hold their knee bent using pressure from your upper arm and body. Stabilise their pelvis with your right hand and draw the left leg back into extension at the hip while maintaining knee flexion.

Variations

Reduce the amount of hip flexion but increase the amount of knee flexion to throw the stretch emphasis to the lower portion of the muscle.

Points to note

The normal range of hip extension is 5–10 degrees before the pelvis begins to tip anteriorly. Where anterior pelvic tilt and increasing lumbar lordosis become excessive, have your partner draw up their right knee and hold it. Stabilising the non-stretching (right) leg into hip flexion will posteriorly tilt the pelvis against the anterior tilt force imposed by the extending (left) stretch leg.

Exercise 101 Rectus femoris – prone

Starting position and instructions

Lie on the floor on your front and bend your right knee. Your partner half kneels at your left hip and places one hand in the small of your back and the other beneath your right knee. Your right foot rests on your partner's shoulder. By leaning forwards, your partner presses your right leg into extension at the hip and flexion at the knee while preventing any lumbar movement.

Variations

Increasing the amount of hip extension will emphasise the upper portion of the muscle; reducing hip extension but increasing knee flexion targets the lower portion.

Points to note

Abduction of the hip should be avoided during this exercise as it releases some of the stretch from the rectus femoris.

Exercise 102 Anterior chest and shoulders – prone

Starting position and instructions

Lie on the floor on your front with both hands in the small of your back. Your partner kneels at your head. Grasping your outer elbows, your partner leans back to pull your arms inwards and upwards. This movement stretches the anterior deltoid, pectoral and biceps muscles.

Variations

Pressing the elbows closer together, or leaving them further apart, will alter the exact site of the stretch.

Points to note

As with all partner stretches, the subject receiving the stretch must give feedback to lead the movement at all times. As the arm is pulled back (extension), the ball of the shoulder socket (head of the humerus) moves forwards. If you have had a shoulder dislocation, this movement should not be practised, as it can overstretch the already lax anterior structures of the joint.

Exercise 103 Shoulder distraction – lying

Starting position and instructions

Begin with your partner/client lying on a gym bench or treatment couch. Hold their left shoulder securely by placing their hand beneath your upper arm and cradling their left arm in the crook of your left arm. Lock the position by placing your right hand on top of their arm and gripping with your right hand. Grip your right upper arm with your left hand (4-lock position). Gradually lean backwards to impart a distraction force on their arm. Hold the position for 30 seconds and then release.

Variations

Perform an oscillation action (longitudinal joint mobilisation) by gently distracting and then releasing their arm in a rhythmic fashion for 20–30 repetitions.

Points to note

Very little force (2–5 lb) is required for this action. The aim is to allow your partner's muscles to relax completely as you apply the distraction force targeted at the joint structures. This action should not be used on an individual with a history of shoulder dislocation unless it is applied by a registered physiotherapist.

Exercise 104 Mobilisation with movement in wall support standing

Variations
Hook a belt around your partners shoulder and pull with the belt rather than your hands.

Points to note
When the shoulder is stiff or has been painful, it may move out of alignment with the ball, catching (impinging) on the edge of the socket. The aim of this action is to keep the ball within the centre of the socket and prevent impingement. Very little force is required, and the amount can be judged by the effect. If the shoulder is painful at the point of maximum overhead stretch, enough force is applied to reduce the pain. If pain increases, or does not reduce, then the technique is not suitable for your partner's shoulder condition.

Starting position and instructions
Your training partner begins by standing facing a wall with their arms stretched overhead, hands resting on the wall. Stand behind your partner and cup your hands around the front of their left shoulder joint. Keeping their arms straight, have your partner bend their knees and push their chest towards the wall to press their shoulder into extension/abduction. As they perform this action, you gently draw their shoulder backwards to keep the ball (head of humerus) of their joint in the centre of the socket (glenoid).

DYNAMIC STRETCHES

11

GUIDELINES FOR DYNAMIC STRETCHING

We saw in chapter 4 that dynamic stretching is simply stretching with movement. It is similar to ballistic stretching as it uses the speed of the body's movement to assist the stretch (as opposed to static stretching, which uses no movement), but dynamic stretching does not involve the bouncing for which ballistic stretching is famous. Dynamic stretching usually uses the body's full range of motion at either single or multiple joints and makes the stretch more functional, as it involves a combination of several different fitness components including stretching, muscle contraction, muscle control and movement rehearsal (skill and timing). The action is therefore specific to the movement patterns involved in sport or daily living, and as such closely follows the *specificity principles* outlined on page 53.

In order to stretch the muscle dynamically the opposing muscle group must contract to instigate the movement. As the stretched muscle is elongated it will store elastic energy (see chapter 1) which will be released as the muscle recoils. The recoil effect takes place in the fascial elements of the muscle, which will be emphasised in chapter 14.

All dynamic stretching exercises should be performed after a warm-up of a sufficient intensity to induce light sweating, such as a brisk walk, static cycling or a gentle jog. Once you are warm, static stretches relevant to the dynamic movement to be used should be practised. For example, an arm swing dynamic stretch should be preceded by overhead reaching. The aim is to take the limb through the full range of motion used in the dynamic stretch.

Initially, all dynamic stretches should be performed while stationary (also called 'in place') and once the exercise is familiar the movement can be performed while moving. Using an arm swing action as an example again, the movement is performed for 5–10 repetitions while standing still. After a brief (30-second) rest, the movement is repeated while walking. This additional movement serves to develop coordination, as you will not be able to simply focus your attention on the arm action alone. Table 11.1 summarises these guidelines.

Key point:

Dynamic stretching uses movement patterns rather than static stretches and therefore can be highly specific to a sports action.

Table 11.1	Guidelines for the practice of dynamic stretching exercises

- Begin with a warm-up that is sufficient to induce mild sweating

- Perform static stretching matched to the body part and range of motion to be used in dynamic stretching

- Perform the dynamic stretch in a slow, controlled manner

- Progress the speed of movement gradually until it matches that to be used in sport

- Perform the dynamic stretch while standing still

- Progress to walking activities

Figure 11.1 Example of combined movement dynamic stretch for kicking

COMBINED MOVEMENTS

In everyday movements, and especially in sport, we rarely perform 'pure' actions such as flexion or extension. These movements are said to be 'single plane' actions as they occur in only one of the three body planes (*see* page 17). In reality, we normally combine the three movement planes and perform actions such as flexion with abduction and rotation. This combination of movements is more demanding in terms of coordination, and so must be practised gradually.

Leg actions, such as kicking, combine actions across the body: flexion with adduction, followed by extension with abduction. In each case the movements may also be combined with medial or lateral rotation. Throwing actions again combine cross-body actions (flexion and adduction) beginning with a 'wind-up' phase of abduction and extension.

Both throwing and kicking will also use trunk actions. For example, a wind-up for a throw will use trunk rotation, lateral flexion and extension towards the extended arm, followed by trunk rotation, lateral flexion and flexion to follow the throwing arm as it goes forwards in front of the body. A kicking action in football will often combine hip flexion and adduction with medial rotation to strike the ball with the inside of the foot. A round house kick in martial arts combines trunk rotation with hip flexion, abduction and medial rotation to strike the target with the front of the foot or shin.

As these actions are complex, they are best trained by performing the actual sport technique but at a lower level and to repetition. For example, the football kick would be performed slowly at a low level, gradually building up speed and intensity as the player progresses. An example of progression to full kicking is shown in figure 11.1.

Exercise 105 Arm swing – forwards

Exercise 106 Arm swing – sideways

Starting position and instructions

Stand with your feet shoulder width apart and knees slightly bent (soft). Swing the left arm upwards and forwards to shoulder level, then allow it to travel back behind the body-line by one or two hand breadths. Pause, and then repeat using the right arm. Once you are confident with the movement, cut out the pause between the movements and practise alternate arm swings as a single continuous motion.

Variations

Both arms can be swung together rather than alternately. However, make sure that you maintain low back alignment as the arms are swung forwards. Do not allow the lower back to hollow excessively (hyperextend) as the arms are taken overhead.

Points to note

The range of motion of the movement should increase progressively. At first, only swing the arm to shoulder level, and with each repetition gradually increase the range of motion until the arm is taken overhead. The rate of progression will be dictated by your fitness level and shoulder flexibility.

Starting position and instructions

Stand with your feet just wider than shoulder width apart and your knees slightly bent (soft). Swing both arms out to the side, allowing the arm to turn (rotate) naturally so that the thumb points towards the ceiling. Lengthen the arm, avoiding any tendency to shrug your shoulders.

Variations

If you have had a shoulder problem, sideways movements (abduction) can be painful. If this applies to you, limit the movement of this stretch by keeping the arm below shoulder level. If you experience no pain and have practised static stretching without problems, slowly increase the range of motion until you can reach overhead and, eventually, touch your hands together.

Points to note

Do not allow your lower back to hollow excessively (hyperextend) as the arms are taken overhead. Maintain your correct back alignment by tightening your abdominal muscles slightly to increase your core stability.

Exercise 107 Arm rotation – alternate

Starting position and instructions

Stand with your feet shoulder width apart and your knees slightly bent (soft). Take your left arm overhead and touch the back of your head with your left hand. Now, take your right hand backwards and place it behind the small of your back. Reverse the movement, alternating between arms. Gradually speed up the movement so that the exercise becomes a smooth, continuous action.

Variations

If you are unable to take your hand behind your head or back, limit the movement by touching only your ear and the outside of your hip. Gradually increase your range of motion using static stretching before you progress the range of the dynamic stretch.

Points to note

Maintain your alignment throughout the movement. As you reach your arm behind your back, do not allow your shoulder to move forwards. As you reach behind your neck, do not hollow your back.

Exercise 108 Wood chop high

Starting position and instructions

Begin standing with your feet hip width apart, hands together. Reach forwards and upwards over your right shoulder at the same time turning to the right to look at your hands. Reach downwards and forwards to waist level, turning your trunk back to face forwards. Reverse the action to reach upwards and backwards taking your hands over your left shoulder and turning your trunk to the left.

Variations

This action can be performed using a high pulley machine or elastic tubing to add resistance.

Points to note

As you reach forwards and upwards and over your shoulder extend your spine slightly, and as you reach forwards and downwards allow your spine to flex slightly.

Exercise 109 Flexion/extension – kneeling

Variations
You can include hip flexion and extension in this action: as you round your spine, draw your right knee towards your forehead. As you arch your spine, straighten your right leg and take it slightly upwards. Repeat the movement with the other leg.

Points to note
If you use the leg variation, make sure that you control the actions throughout, cutting down the momentum of the moving leg. If the leg moves too quickly, the spine will be forced to flex and extend at the end of each sequence by the movement of the leg. This can introduce dangerous loading forces to the lumbar vertebrae (low back bones) in particular.

Starting position and instructions
Kneel down on all fours with your knees hip width apart and your hands shoulder width apart. Your knees should be directly below your hips and your hands directly below your shoulders. Round (flex) your spine and tuck your tail under (posterior pelvic tilt). Pause in this position, then arch (extend) your spine and point your tail to the ceiling (anterior pelvic tilt). Build the action into a single smooth movement.

Exercise 110 Flexion/extension – standing

Starting position and instructions

Stand with your knees hip width apart and slightly bent (soft). Hold on to a vertical pole. Tilt your pelvis backwards, round your shoulders and flex your spine. Pause in this flexed position, then tilt your pelvis forwards, brace your shoulders and extend your spine. Gradually speed up the movement until you are performing a single smooth action.

Variations

When you are confident with the movement, you can dispense with the stick. When you do this, the exercise works your sense of balance (proprioception) harder. However, make sure that you avoid too much body sway when you do this.

Points to note

Depending on your posture type (*see* pages 77–83) you may find either flexion or extension easier. If this is the case, do not force the stiff movement with dynamic stretching. Instead, develop your flexibility using static stretching, and then maintain it with dynamic stretching.

Exercise 111 Lateral flexion – standing

Starting position and instructions

Stand with your feet one and a half times shoulder width apart and place your hands on your hips. Bend to the left, taking your weight on your left arm. Stand up straight again and then bend to the right, taking your weight on your right arm.

Variations

Once you are confident with the movement, you can perform the action with your arms by your sides. This increases the work of the trunk muscles as they now have to support your full bodyweight. Finally, you can increase the stretch by reaching overhead. As you bend to the left, reach overhead (and slightly to the left) with your right hand. Reverse the action using the left hand as you bend to the right.

Points to note

Asymmetry with this movement is common as many people have a greater degree of flexion to one side than the other. If this is the case, develop your flexibility using the supported side bend (hands on your hips) rather than reaching overhead. Once you have an equal range of motion on both sides, you can progress to the overhead reach action.

Exercise 112 Rotation - standing

Exercise 113 Forward bend

Starting position and instructions

Stand with your feet shoulder width apart and your knees slightly bent (soft). Your arms should be held slightly away from your body. Turn your body to the left, bringing your right arm round in front of you and pointing your hand to the left. At the same time, take your left hand behind you, pointing your hand to the right. Reverse the action.

Variations

You can reduce the forces on the spine by performing the action with your hands on your hips. In this case, the elbows lead the movement and some of your bodyweight is taken through your hips.

Points to note

Make sure that your arms lead the movement, but do not allow them to swing vigorously to force you further into rotation.

Starting position and instructions

Begin standing with your feet hip width apart. Keeping your arms straight, reach them forwards and upwards above your head, arching your back slightly and looking up at your hands. In a smooth continuous action reach your arms forwards and downwards bending your spine and looking at your hands as you do so.

Variations

To reduce the stretch on the hamstrings where these muscles are very tight, slightly bend (soften) your knees throughout the action.

Points to note

In the forward reaching position the back fascia is placed on stretch. This can be increased by maintaining the forward bend position for 5–10 seconds and loosely folding your arms to allow your elbows to reach downwards and forwards. Relax your head to look between your legs rather than downwards at the floor, so that your neck remains in line with the rest of your spine.

Exercise **114** Wood chop low

Starting position and instructions

Begin with your feet slightly wider than hip width apart, hands clasped together. Turn to your right and at the same time reach your hands up and across your right shoulder. Look at your hands throughout the movement, and draw your arms down and forwards turning your trunk to the left as you do so. Take your hands past your left knee to mid-shin level. Perform 5 repetitions of this action, and then reverse the movement reaching from a high left point to low right point.

Variations

This action can be performed using resistance with a high pulling machine or elastic tubing.

Points to note

This is a continuous motion involving several body parts. As the arms and shoulders move the trunk should mimic the movement going from extension as the arms are reached up and backwards, to flexion as the arms reach forwards and downwards. Throughout the movement the legs follow the action, moving into extension as the arms are raised, and into flexion as the arms are lowered.

Exercise **115** Rotation – lying

Starting position and instructions

Lie on your back with your knees bent and feet flat. Keep your arms out to your sides at an angle of 90 degrees to your body. Allow your knees to slowly lower to one side, twisting your trunk as they do so. Pause in the lower position as your knee touches the mat and then pull your legs back up. Repeat to each side.

Variations

If you lift your feet up from the mat so that your knees are directly above your hips, the emphasis is changed to strength throughout the movement. Rather than placing your arms on the mat to support your upper body, you can move your arms in the opposite direction to your legs (knees to the right, arms to the left), which places a greater stretch on the thoracic spine.

Points to note

As the knee is lowered on to the mat, ensure that you keep the action under control. Do not allow your knees to drop, forcing your spine into a rotation range that may be inappropriate. If you find the rotation range too great, allow your knees to lower on to a cushion or block rather than all the way down on to the mat.

Exercise 116 Cervical rotation

Starting position and instructions

Sit on a chair or gym bench with your spine correctly aligned. Sit up tall and draw your chin in slightly. Relax your shoulders and avoid the tendency to shrug them. Loosely fold your arms on your lap or let them hang by the sides to support their weight and assist in shoulder relaxation. Keep your shoulders square, look to your left as far as is comfortable, pause in this rotated position and then look to your right. Repeat the action 5 times, making sure that you pause at each side to avoid feeling dizzy. With each repetition, try to gradually increase your range of motion until your chin passes over your collarbone (clavicle).

Variations

As you twist, you may find that your neck moves into flexion or extension; this means that the rotation movement is not a single pure movement, but is combined with flexion/extension. To avoid this, hold a stick or ruler in front of you just below your nose. As you practise the movement, make sure that your nose does not move away from the ruler (neck extension) or touch the ruler (neck flexion).

Points to note

It is common to suffer asymmetry (where one side of the body is different from the other) in the cervical spine. If you notice that the rotation to one side is less than that to the other side, do not force the movement on the stiff side.

Exercise 117 Leg swing – sideways

Starting position and instructions

Stand facing a piece of gym equipment with your feet hip width apart. Hold on to the apparatus with both hands. Shift your pelvis to the left to take your whole weight onto your left leg and unload your right. Swing your right leg out to the side and then inwards and in front of the left leg (abduction and adduction). Start by swinging outwards to shin level, then knee level and finally, hip level. As you swing your leg, do not allow your trunk to twist.

Variations

Pointing your toes to the ceiling combines hip abduction with lateral rotation. Pointing your heel to the ceiling (toes to the floor) combines abduction with medial rotation. Use a combination of both actions to balance your training programme unless your medial rotators are especially long, in which case the lateral rotation movement alone should be emphasised.

Points to note

In order to unload the swinging leg, you must transfer your bodyweight over the other (weight-bearing) leg. This should be achieved by shifting the pelvis over the weight-bearing leg. However, if you lack hip control and hip stability, you may find that you simply tip your spine sideways (lateral flexion of the trunk). Try to avoid this action by keeping your spine upright and your pelvis level.

Exercise 118 Leg swing – forwards and backwards

Exercise 119 Knee to elbow

Starting position and instructions

Stand with your feet shoulder width apart. Hold on to a bar or the frame of a piece of gym apparatus at your right side for balance. Swing your left leg forwards and upwards into flexion, first to shin level, then to waist level and eventually to chest level. Progress the range of motion as you feel comfortable, being careful not to overstretch.

As the limb goes backwards, maintain your low back alignment; do not allow your back to hollow excessively (hyperextend).

Variations

Keeping the leg straight places the stretch on the single joint hip flexors (iliopsoas) and the extensors. Allowing the knee to bend as though kicking the backside will stretch the rectus femoris as well.

Points to note

Ensure, therefore, that the action is controlled throughout the whole range of movement. Do not allow the momentum to pull you into a range that you would not usually use.

Starting position and instructions

Stand with your feet shoulder width apart and your arms held slightly abducted with your forearms horizontal. Bring your right knee up to touch your right elbow, lower the leg and then repeat, this time bringing your left knee to your left elbow.

Variations

You can also use a diagonal pattern, taking the right knee to the left elbow and vice versa. The movement can be progressed to a knee-to-elbow walk by placing the foot forwards rather than directly downwards and moving along in a high-knee walk.

Points to note

Make sure that you pull your knee up to your elbow rather than bending forwards and taking your elbow down to your knee. Aim to keep your trunk upright and your spine vertical throughout the exercise.

Exercise 120 Lunge walk

Starting position and instructions

Stand with your feet shoulder width apart and your hands by your sides. Step forwards with your left leg in a lunging action, placing your foot flat on the floor. Aim to have your knee pass beyond your foot and your thigh horizontal. Step back so that your feet are again shoulder width apart and repeat the movement with your right leg. Once you have performed 5 repetitions on each leg, rest for 30–60 seconds. Then step forwards with your left leg into a lunge, press yourself back up again and then step forwards with the right, aiming to move along in a deep 'walking' action.

Variations

Initially, you perform the lunge walk with your arms by your sides. However, the balance of the movement is made easier if you extend your arms out sideways in a 'T' position. If you find the lunge is too hard on your legs, place one hand on the thigh of the forward lunging leg and press on it to bring yourself back up to standing.

Points to note

The downward movement of the lunge must be controlled; take care not to 'fall' into the position. In addition, make sure that you keep your trunk upright, avoiding the temptation to lean forwards by flexing the trunk on the hip. Fix your eyes on a distant point to help you with this.

Exercise 121 Calf stretch – with a band

Exercise 122 Calf stretch – sprint start

Starting position and instructions

Sit on a mat with your legs straight out in front of you. Place a rolled towel beneath your calf muscles to allow free movement of your heels. Pull your feet towards you, then point them away from you.

Variations

This exercise can also be performed by hooking an exercise band around the ball of your feet. Allow the band to pull your feet upwards (dorsiflexion), then point your toes against the resistance of the band. You can perform the stretch one leg at a time if this feels more comfortable. Hooking the band around your toes rather than the ball of your foot will also place the stretch on the deep toe flexors as well as the calf.

Points to note

There are two main calf muscles: the soleus, which acts over the ankle alone; and the gastrocnemius, which acts over both the ankle and the knee. To target the gastrocnemius muscle (the larger of the two), perform the action with your knees straight. To work the soleus muscle, perform the movement with your knees slightly bent.

Starting position and instructions

Stand in a lunge position with your right leg back and your left leg forwards, with your weight over your front leg. Place the toes of your back foot on the ground and gradually take your weight backwards, forcing your heel on to the ground as you do so. Pause, then use the calf strength of your back leg to 'flick' you forwards as though exploding out of the blocks from a sprint start. Repeat the exercise 5 times with the right leg back, then reverse the movement.

Variations

Placing your back leg further back will increase the intensity of the stretch; taking your leg further forwards will reduce it. You can emphasise the power aspect of this movement rather than the stretch by taking more weight on to your back leg and jumping slightly as you flick yourself forwards.

Points to note

Make sure that you build the range of motion progressively. Start with your feet quite close together and gradually move your back leg further backwards as your confidence in the movement grows.

STRETCHING
// USING EQUIPMENT

12

Many exercises involve equipment, with machines and free weights being perhaps the most commonly used. However, equipment can be useful in stretching, which is traditionally an exercise type performed with bodyweight and limb loading alone. Equipment can offer significant advantages for maintaining alignment and for providing overload to the tissues. In this chapter we will look at several stretching exercises using equipment, but bear in mind many exercises may be modified with equipment at some stage in their performance. Where this is the case the equipment is mentioned under *variations* and *points to note* in the general stretching chapters.

Exercise 123 Knee extension – with a towel

Starting position and instructions
Lie on the floor with the left leg straight and flex the right knee and hip to 90 degrees. Hook a folded towel around your right foot, holding one end of the towel in each hand. Rest your upper arms on the mat and attempt to straighten your leg by pushing your foot into the towel. Do not allow your arms to straighten, and keep the hip, knee and foot in a straight line.

Variations
Instead of a towel, use an exercise band or yoga belt. Make sure that the band is positioned in the centre of the foot rather than on the toes to guard against slipping.

Points to note
Fastening the towel over your toes will pull the toes towards you. Combining this movement with flexion of the neck will throw stress on to the neural tissues and sciatic nerve and away from the hamstrings (*see* Stretching the nerves, chapter 13).

Exercise 124 Lying hamstring stretch – with a belt

Starting position and instructions

Begin lying on your back on the floor, and fasten a yoga belt around the centre of your right foot. Lift your right leg to 90 degrees keeping it straight, and wind the yoga belt around your gripped hands. Take the slack up from the belt and, keeping your arms straight, reach overhead to draw your straight leg into further flexion. At your full range, maintain the static stretch for 20–30 seconds.

Variations

Moving the arms inwards will draw the leg into flexion and adduction, while moving the arms outwards will draw it into flexion and abduction. Both give a slightly different emphasis to the muscle stretch.

Points to note

This is an intense stretch and you must move into it gradually. The straight leg position places a stretching force on both the hamstrings and the sciatic nerve. Where you feel pins and needles into your foot the nerve is stimulated (neural tension – *see* chapter 13). Pointing the toes and keeping the head resting on the floor reduces tension on the sciatic nerve, while dorsiflexing the foot and flexing the neck increases it.

Exercise 125 Rectus femoris – lying

Starting position and instructions

Lie on the floor on your front and bend your right knee. Loop a towel or yoga belt around your right ankle and pull your knee into flexion, drawing your heel towards your buttock. Keep your knee in line with your hip, avoiding the tendency to move the knee outward (hip abduction).

Variations

Place your knee on a block, forcing the hip into extension. This emphasises the upper portion of the muscle.

Points to note

Make sure you stretch both the upper and lower portions of the muscle for the same number of repetitions.

Exercise 126 Side flexion – over a roll

Starting position and instructions

Roll up a bath towel to form a 15–20 cm thick roll. Lie on your side on a mat and place the roll under the side of your trunk, between the rim of your pelvis and your lower ribs. Allow your pelvis and hips to sink down into the mat and reach your upper arm over your head to try to touch the mat. Hold the stretch for 20–30 seconds, breathing normally.

Variations

Crossing your legs and bringing your top leg forwards will allow your pelvis to tip further sideways, increasing the intensity of the stretch. A 15 cm foam roller may be used in place of the towel, but it is firmer and some people find it less comfortable.

Points to note

This stretch targets the side flexors of the trunk (obliques and quadratus lumborum) and the latissimus dorsi. To isolate the trunk, keep your arm at your side and do not reach overhead.

Exercise 127 Whole back extension – over a gym ball

Starting position and instructions

Sit on a gym ball with your knees and hips bent to 90 degrees. Your feet should be wider than shoulder width apart and flat on the floor. Walk your feet forwards so that the gym ball rolls under your back and stop when it lies between your shoulder blades. Straighten your arms and reach over your head and back towards the floor, allowing your hips to drop down towards the floor at the same time.

Variations

By adjusting the position of the gym ball, you can determine which area of your spine receives the greatest stretch.

Points to note

This is an extreme stretch, but is quite comfortable to hold as the whole of the spine is supported. If you find the stretch too difficult, deflate the gym ball slightly so that it is flatter and more squashy. The flatter contour of the ball will reduce the intensity of the stretch.

Exercise 128 Thoracic spine – over a roll

Exercise 129 Overhead reach – using a belt

Starting position and instructions

Lie flat on the floor on your back with your knees bent and feet flat. Have your training partner place a rolled towel beneath your thoracic spine so that the towel runs perpendicular to your spine. Straighten your arms and grip your hands together loosely. Breathe in and raise your arms overhead, trying to touch the mat behind you. As you do so, allow your thoracic spine to be stretched over the towel. Do not lift your spine off the mat.

Variations

Altering the position of the towel will change the focus of the movement. Shuffling up and down will enable you to place the towel at the exact point of stiffness in the thoracic spine. If you find that the towel is uncomfortable, use two small towels and place them end-to-end so that there is a 2 cm gap between them. Place this gap beneath the spinous processes of your back.

Points to note

The exercise can be performed with the legs straight to lengthen the spine along its entire span. However, with the legs straight it is easy to arch the lower back, which in turn takes some of the stretch away from the thoracic spine. If the legs are kept straight, ensure that the hollow beneath the lower back (lumbar lordosis) does not increase.

Starting position and instructions

Begin by fastening a yoga belt around your upper arms, with your arms shoulder width apart. Stand with your feet together and reach overhead keeping your arms straight, palms facing together. Press your straight arms outwards into the resistance of the belt to activate your arm and shoulder muscles as you reach upwards. Ensure that you maintain good spinal alignment and avoid increasing the hollow in your lumbar spine (lumbar lordosis).

Variations

Beginning with your arms wider (1½ or 2 times shoulder width) reduces the abduction range at the shoulder and makes the movement easier. However, this reduced abduction also reduces the stretching effect on the latissimus dorsi muscle.

Points to note

By activating the arm muscles as you press into the belt, tactile cueing is increased enabling you to maintain better upper body alignment.

Exercise 130 Spinal rotation – using a stick

Exercise 131 Lateral flexion – using a stick

Starting position and instructions

Sit astride a bench with a stick across your shoulders. Grip the ends of the stick and twist your trunk to the left, pressing your left elbow backwards and your right elbow forwards. This movement stretches the oblique abdominals.

Variations

Reaching your hands above your head before beginning the stretch will pull harder on the thoracolumbar fascia.

Points to note

This exercise must be performed slowly, with a hold at the end to avoid building up potentially damaging momentum. If your shoulder flexibility does not permit you to place the stick across your shoulders, hold it on the front of the chest at the level of the upper part of your breastbone.

Starting position and instructions

Sit on a stool or astride a bench with a stick across your shoulders. Grip the ends of the stick and laterally flex to the left, moving the stick upwards towards the ceiling. This movement stretches the external oblique and quadratus lumborum on the right-hand side of the body.

Variations

A towel can be used instead of the stick if your shoulder is not flexible enough to allow the stick to be placed behind your neck. Alternatively, hold the stick on your chest at the level of the upper part of your breastbone.

Points to note

Pure lateral flexion should be used rather than combining it with flexion or rotation. In addition, the pivot point of the movement should be at the level of the breastbone (sternum) rather than at the waist. Pivoting around the breastbone keeps the body upright, while pivoting around the waist causes the body to lean sideways.

Exercise **132** Upper trapezius – with a band

Starting position and instructions
Stand of the floor holding a band in both hands. Place the band beneath your feet and stand upright. Shrug your shoulders against the resistance of the band, then let the band draw your shoulders down and slightly backwards.

Variations
A heavier-resistance band can be used for a greater stretch.

Points to note
The emphasis should be on the stretch, so shrug the shoulders for two counts and allow four counts for the band to stretch the shoulders downwards. Make sure that you maintain your spinal alignment throughout this movement; do not allow the band to pull you down into flexion.

Exercise **133** Combined shoulder rotation – using a towel

Starting position and instructions
Grasp a towel behind your back with your right arm placed behind your neck and your left arm in the small of your back. Move your arms up and down to lift and lower the towel vertically.

Variations
A broom handle can be used instead of the towel, or, if you are very flexible, you may be able to grasp your hands together. If you perform the exercise sitting or kneeling on the floor, bending the trunk slightly will increase the intensity of the stretch by pressing the lower arm further backwards.

Points to note
Asymmetry in shoulder rotation is common, so the range of motion may differ when the arm placement changes.

Exercise 134 Back flexion – on a gym ball

Starting position and instructions
Sit on a gym ball large enough to allow your hips to be slightly above your knees, keeping your knees just wider than shoulder width apart. As you sit, you are on your sitting bones (ischial tuberosities). Tilt your pelvis backwards so that you are sitting more on your tailbone and allow your lower back to bend (flex). Pause in this stretched position, then tilt your pelvis forwards so that you are sitting on your pubic bone, a little like riding a horse.

Variations
You can involve the whole spine in the stretch by bending to look at your umbilicus (belly button) as you tilt your pelvis backwards to sit on your tail. As you tilt your pelvis forwards to sit on your pubic bone, look upwards towards the ceiling and arch (hollow) the whole of your back.

Points to note
Try to avoid 'body sway' when performing the movement, as it makes you less stable on the ball. The aim should be to keep your shoulders over the top of your hips throughout. Placing your hands on your knees will aid your balance; having them out to the sides makes the balance more difficult. If you find that you wobble noticeably during the movement, place a chair or gym bench in front of you and hold on to that as you move.

Exercise 135 External shoulder rotation – using a stick

Starting position and instructions
Grip a bar above your head. Lower your arms so that the bar passes behind your neck, hold the position and then release. This movement stretches the medial rotators of the shoulder (subscapularis, deltoid, latissimus dorsi and pectoralis major).

Variations
A towel can be used instead of the bar, provided that you keep the towel taut.

Points to note
Asymmetry in rotation is common, so one arm may be able to drop lower than the other.

Exercise 136 Forearm pronation and supination – using a stick

Exercise 137 Wrist extensors – on a table

Starting position and instructions

Flex your right elbow and turn your forearm so that your palm faces upwards. Gripping a stick in your right hand, support your forearm in your cupped left hand. Pronate and supinate your right forearm, using the weight of the stick as overpressure.

Variations

Using a lighter or heavier stick will change the intensity of the stretch.

Points to note

Holding the stretch at the end of the range of motion will increase the overload.

Starting position and instructions

Place your right hand palm-down at the edge of a low table and place your left hand on top of your right so that your thumb is level with your wrist crease. Press the right forearm down into the vertical position, pressing your right wrist into extension. Use the weight from your left hand to keep the heel of your right hand on the table.

Variations

Altering the height of the table will vary the range of motion of the wrist.

Points to note

Where a single intercarpel joint is stiff, the movement can be localised by firmly pressing the thumb of the left hand into the wrist crease of the right hand.

STRETCHING THE NERVES

13

Stretching exercises are generally said to affect the muscles, with less effect on the joint tissues. However, an important structure that may be affected when performing stretching exercises is the nervous system.

Any exercise that moves a limb will have an impact on the nerves as well as the muscles, and these effects must be considered when giving stretching exercises. As a limb is bent or straightened, the nerves must adapt. With elbow flexion, for example, the ulnar nerve is stretched while the radial and median nerves are shortened. In fact, from fully bending the elbow and wrist to fully straightening them, nerves can change their length by as much as 20 per cent. Any stretching exercise we perform will have effects on the nerves and, through them, on other tissues seemingly unconnected to the body part we are using.

STRUCTURE OF THE NERVOUS SYSTEM

The nervous system can be visualised as an 'H' turned on its side, with the central bar of the 'H' being the spinal cord and the crossbars the nerves to the arms and legs. This structure is often divided into the central nervous system (CNS) – consisting of the brain and spinal cord – and the peripheral nervous system – consisting

> **Key point:**
>
> In normal movements, nerves may stretch (lengthen) by up to 20 per cent.

of the nerves in the legs and arms. However, this division is misleading, because structurally many of the tissues within the nervous system are connected with each other, and the chemical reactions and electrical impulses within the nervous system travel its entire length. The nervous system can, therefore, be considered as a 'continuous tissue tract', a little like a single piece of string looping through the spine and limbs. Any tension (pulling) on one part will be transmitted throughout the whole structure and will have effects at points distant to the original site of disruption.

There are two types of nerve cells in nervous tissue: those that carry electrical nerve impulses (neurons), and those that protect and support the delicate conducting structures of the nervous system (neuroglial cells). In the limbs, the peripheral nervous system is made up of neurons, which have a cell body and long arms stretching out into the limb (see fig 13.1). The cell body is located close to the spine, with the cell's arm stretching the whole length of the limb. For example, a single nerve cell may stretch from the lumbar spine along the whole length of the leg to the big toe! The cell's arm (axon) is covered with an insulating material called myelin, which is produced from the neuroglial cells. The structure of the axon can be compared to an electrical cable of copper wire covered with insulating rubber. The nerve cells are grouped into bundles (fascicles) and the bundles are covered by a variety of membranes, the innermost being the endoneurium.

In the central nervous system, the brain connects to the spinal cord at the base of the skull, and from the cord 'nerve roots' arise at 'T' junctions.

Several nerve roots may come together to form a peripheral nerve travelling into the limbs. The cord, nerve root and peripheral nerve each have a protective covering, but that of the nerve root is different from the other two structures. In addition, the point at which the nerve root leaves the spinal cord is very close to the vertebral bones themselves, so the space is restricted. The combination of restricted space and poorer protection leaves the nerve root exposed to stress from certain movements and back injuries.

Attached alongside the spinal cord is the autonomic nervous system (part of the peripheral nervous system and consisting of sympathetic and parasympathetic parts), which provides the nervous control of the internal body environment, regulating, for example, heart rate and blood pressure. In addition, it controls aspects of the skin such as sweating and skin blood flow. Involvement of the autonomic nervous system in injury may, for example, cause whiteness in the skin with feelings of hot and cold, and sweating.

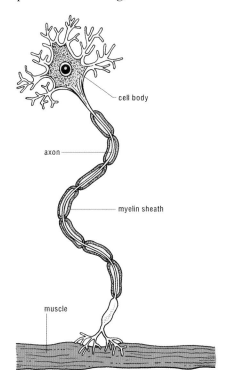

Figure 13.1 Structure of a nerve cell

cell body

axon

myelin sheath

muscle

> **Key point:**
>
> The nerves of the limbs (arms and legs) join the spinal cord via the nerve roots.

BIOMECHANICS OF THE NERVOUS SYSTEM

When nerves are stretched, they can do only one of two things: they can lengthen or 'give' and slide, or they can develop tension. Tension development is in the form of compression of the tissues and fluids contained in the nerve sheaths.

Movement of the nervous system may occur as a whole (gross movement), as in the case of a nerve sliding through a bony tunnel on the outside of the elbow. This movement may also be quite large: in the case of the spinal cord moving from full extension to full flexion, the cord can lengthen by nearly 10 cm, most of the movement being in the cervical and lumbar regions with little movement in the thoracic spine. With traction used by physiotherapists, a 5 kg stretching force can elongate the cervical spine by 10 mm and therefore stretch the spinal cord. Compression caused by carrying heavy weights will similarly compress the spine.

The nervous system, however, does not move consistently along its whole length as tension points occur (*see* fig 13.2). These are at the level of the sixth cervical vertebra (C6), the sixth thoracic vertebra (T6), and the fourth lumbar vertebra (L4). With flexion, tethering (attachment) at these points means the spinal cord will be stretched towards the neck and lumbar spine, but away from the thoracic spine.

Parts of the nervous system can also move in relation to others, a process known as intraneural movement. For example, the spinal cord can slide within its containing sheath (dura mater), one nerve fibre within a bundle can move in relation to another, or an individual fibre can move in relation to its own sheath. In lateral flexion of the spine, the convex side of the spinal cord stretches in relation to the other, the difference in length being as much as 15 per cent.

In the case of gross movement, an injury that causes bruising or swelling over a region of the body may cause the nerve passing through this region to become adhered to other tissues. These types of injuries can range from bruising from a simple muscle pull affecting a nerve as it passes through the muscle – for example the sciatic nerve in relation to the hamstrings – to calluses from a healing bone growing around the nerve – as in the case of the ulna nerve travelling around the outside of the elbow. These types of tethering will lead to nerve irritation and/or pain whenever the region is placed on stretch until the nerve breaks free. Intraneural movement may be limited if a crush injury causes swelling and scarring to regions of the nerve itself. If the individual nerve fibres within a bundle can no longer slide in relation to each other as a nerve is stretched around a corner, for example when bending the knee, tension and pain may result.

VULNERABLE AREAS OF THE NERVOUS SYSTEM

Nerves have several vulnerable areas (*see* fig 13.3).

ANATOMICAL TUNNELS

These are tunnels formed through or around bone or soft tissues that have relatively rigid walls and are therefore unyielding. Excessive movement may cause a build-up of friction, especially in the presence of swelling within the tunnel from a minor injury. An example of a nerve tunnel is the median nerve travelling through the tunnel made by the small wrist (carpal) bones. This area, called the carpel tunnel, can give rise to 'carpal tunnel syndrome', a condition in which pressure on the medial nerve as it travels into the wrist gives aching and tingling sensations in the hand.

Figure 13.2 Tension points in the nervous system

Key point:

Following any injury that causes bruising and swelling, nerves may be stuck down anatomical tunnels (tethered) by clotted fluid.

NERVE BRANCHES

A nerve is at risk when it branches, especially when this branching construction forms an acute angle. An example of this configuration is the digital nerve branching into the fourth and fifth toes. Pressure on this area through incorrect footwear can cause tissue tension and the development of a small cyst called a digital neuroma. This painful condition gives a burning sensation in the fourth and fifth toes due to nerve pressure.

FIXATION POINTS

The fixation points of the nervous system will not allow the normal sliding of nerves against underlying tissues and pressure near these points will be poorly tolerated. An example of a fixation point is at the head of the fibula bone where the common peroneal nerve wraps itself around it. Damage to this area is common, for example from a direct blow from a football boot or hockey ball. The resultant swelling and scarring tethers the nerve, giving symptoms of injury.

FRICTION POINTS

At certain points the nerves pass over, or close to, unyielding structures. Any tension will cause the nerve to give, but this will be limited. An example is where the brachial nerves extend from the cervical spine and pass over the first rib before travelling into the arm. Carrying heavy shopping bags can pull the nerves down on to the rib, giving pain and tingling in the whole arm (brachial neuralgia).

TENSION POINTS

The classic tension points of the nervous system (*see* fig 13.2) will cause the movement direction of the nerves to change, and are potential areas of concern. The sixth thoracic vertebra and the posterior aspect of the knee are examples, and these points are frequently a source of neural pain when stretching (*see* table 13.1).

EFFECTS OF STRETCHING THE NERVOUS SYSTEM

Stretching a nerve has many effects: some that aid healing, and some that can be damaging.

HEALING EFFECTS

After an injury that causes swelling, a nerve stretch will move the nerve past the swollen area preventing the clotted swelling from sticking (adhering) to the nerve. In addition, any swelling within the nerve between its individual fibres may also be dispersed by pressure changes brought about through rhythmic stretching. Following

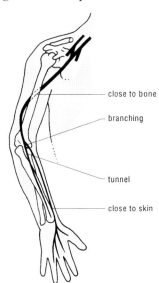

Figure 13.3 Vulnerable areas of a typical nerve

close to bone

branching

tunnel

close to skin

Table 13.1	Vulnerable areas of the nervous system
Anatomical tunnels	A tunnel has relatively rigid, unyielding walls and, therefore, the nerve is susceptible to pressure, e.g. median nerve travelling through the wrist (carpel tunnel).
Nerve branches	When a nerve branches at an acute angle its gliding mechanism is reduced. There is, therefore, less movement available to it, e.g. digital nerve branching into the fourth and fifth toes.
Fixation points	Fixation points are less yielding and nerves are more likely to be injured by tension at these points, e.g. common peroneal nerve wrapping around the head of the fibula.
Friction points	Where a nerve passes close to unyielding tissues, there is an increased likelihood of pressure, e.g. brachial plexus nerves passing over the first rib.
Tension points	Points where the direction of neural movement is reversed, e.g. sixth thoracic vertebra and posterior aspect of the knee.

chronic injury, a nerve may become tethered to underlying structures: stretching can break the nerve free of its binding scar tissue and allow nerve impulses to pass unimpeded once more. Rhythmic movement will also improve the blood supply to the nerve, and with it the amount of oxygen reaching the nervous tissue. In addition, the transport system within the nerve, called axonal transport, will be improved by movement and reduced by prolonged inactivity.

Key point:

Rhythmic stretching can release a tethered nerve and improve the transport system within the nerve.

DAMAGING EFFECTS
Repeated stretching

As with muscle and bone, the physical stresses involved with repeated stretching will cause minor injury (microtrauma), which will encourage the tissue to adapt and become stronger. However, caution is necessary with repeated microtrauma: if the degree of physical stress exceeds the capacity of the nerve (or any tissue) to adapt, tissue breakdown and injury may result.

Continuous stretching

When a nerve is stretched continuously, for example by poor posture, its blood flow may be impaired. As the stretch is placed on, the blood vessels supplying the nerve become thinner. With just 8 per cent lengthening of the nerve, blood flow to the nerve begins to reduce substantially, and when the nerve is stretched by 15 per cent, the blood flow is completely cut off. If this happens only once, or if the nerve is released, allowed to recover, and then stretched again, no problem will arise.

However, prolonged blood flow reduction can cause problems. Initially, the reduction in blood flow causes the blood within the vessels to stagnate, and all the oxygen within it is rapidly used up. This oxygen starvation is known as hypoxia, and the result is often pain and pins and needles that reduces when the blood flow is reinstated. Crossing the legs for prolonged periods in the cinema is a good example of neural hypoxia. When the legs are released, a shower of pins and needles ensues, followed by warmth and a return of normal sensation when full oxygen levels are rebuilt. If the hypoxia remains, however, permanent injury may result: the lining of the small blood capillaries can become damaged and proteins can leak out into the surrounding area, causing a change in fluid pressure leading to local swelling, which being unable to escape, spreads along the length of the nerve. The swelling may eventually clot, causing a build-up of scar tissue within the area. The scarring will often stick to surrounding structures, preventing the nerve from sliding properly with everyday movements and causing friction as the nerve passes through tunnels and across other structures. More damage and nerve irritation occurs and pain is the inevitable result. In this way, minimal damage is exacerbated and a minor problem in one area spreads, causing symptoms in other body parts.

Prolonged stretching

Stretching over a prolonged period may actually cause the nerve to lengthen. Hamstring stretching, for example, may cause the sciatic nerve to lengthen permanently.

Key point:

Poor posture can place continuous stress on a nerve, reducing its blood supply and starving it of oxygen.

STRETCHING EXERCISE FOR NERVES

When targeting nerves with a stretching programme we use two techniques, sliding and tensioning. Nerve sliding is caused by movement in a stretched position (dynamic stretch) while tensioning uses a constant stretch action (static stretch).

NERVE TENSIONING

Nerve tensioning involves combining movement of several joints at the same time, to stretch the nerve to the point of movement limitation or pain onset, and holding this action for 20–40 seconds.

A number of positions will cause tension build-up in the nervous tissue. Sometimes these positions are similar to classic stretches, and on other occasions they add subtle changes to a movement to apply a further stretch. In all cases, it must be remembered that nerves are delicate structures that must be treated with respect. Any nerve stretch may cause not just a feeling of tightness and aching, but pins and needles as well. This indicates that a stretch is working, but is too harsh. If this occurs, the stretch should be released slightly so that the feeling is just short of producing pins and needles. Over time, as the nerve stretches further, the point at which pins and needles occurs will move further away as the range of motion increases. Most of the stretches detailed below are combinations of several movements. When a nerve is adhered and causing problems, the stretch should begin with the distal movement, away from the tight structures. For example, if a combination of trunk flexion, straightening the leg and pulling the foot up (see the classic slump, exercise 138, overleaf) causes problems in someone who is recovering from low back pain, the stretch should be released by allowing the knee to bend and the back to straighten slightly. Further stretch is gradually added by first pulling the foot up into dorsiflexion and then straightening the knee. Only at the last moment should the hip be flexed or the trunk bent further – a sliding technique may also be used (see below).

After stretching, nervous tissue will need to recover in the same way that a muscle does. Remember that stretching a nerve reduces its blood flow, so adequate recovery must be allowed for. For this reason, nerve stretches should only be practised on alternate days, and a gentle warmth and general feeling of stretch is all that is required. Nerve stretches that cause pain are too extreme.

NERVE SLIDING

Nerve sliding (gliding) involves movement of at least two joints with one lengthening the nerve and the other shortening it. The combination of lengthening and shortening maintains the overall nerve length and unloads the nerve, and improves nerve motility. Practically, the combination is movement to the distal tissues (limb) while maintaining the position of the proximal tissue (spine) and then reversing the sequence and moving the proximal tissues while keeping the distal tissue still. Sustained nerve tension increases intraneural pressure and reduces local blood flow, which may lead to local oedema and can trigger spontaneous local nerve activity (ectopic discharge) from sensitive nerves, increasing a subject's pain. Sliding, by maintaining overall nerve length may be seen as a gentler technique. The exercise position is the same, but the technique of execution different.

Exercise 138 The classic slump

Starting position and instructions

Sit on a stool and link your arms behind your back. Gently flex your spine, beginning with your neck. At the same time straighten one of your legs, moving your foot up and your leg into a horizontal position.

Variations

Components of this action may be used individually at first, then built up into a full sequence. If one leg is very tight, keep that knee bent and gradually work towards straightening it, easing into the tightness but not forcing the movement. This can be achieved by placing the tight leg on top of the other and using the lower leg to provide a passive stretch while the upper leg relaxes. Alternatively, support the foot of the tight leg on the floor by placing it on a shiny piece of paper. With the weight of the leg taken through the floor, slide the foot forwards and backwards, again gradually working towards the fully extended position.

Points to note

This action stretches the whole of the nervous system, affecting the spinal cord, upper limb nerves and lower limb nerves of the straightened leg. As soon as you feel any tingling or resistance to the stretch, release the movement by flexing the leg slightly. Maintain this position for 20–30 seconds and then release. For the next repetition, again go just short of the point of pain/tingling, hoping to push this point further away, enabling you to straighten your leg further.

Exercise 139 Nerve sliding in slump position

Starting position and instructions

Begin in the classic slump position described above, ensuring that your foot is clear of the floor. Keep your spine flexed throughout the exercise and bend (flex) your neck to bring your head down to your breastbone (sternum) and at the same time keep your knee bent and point your toes and foot (plantarflexion). Straighten your knee and draw your foot and toes towards you (ankle dorsiflexion and toe flexion and at the same time look up at the ceiling (cervical extension). Repeat the action rhythmically for 10 repetitions.

Variations

Where there is a high degree of tightness, or where pain occurs, the exercise can be performed in two parts. First, keep the head still and move the leg, and second, keep the leg still and move the head. When both actions are pain free they may be combined.

Points to note

This action is also called a seated straight leg slider by physiotherapists.

The straight leg sliding technique has been shown to increase range of motion of the hamstring muscles (measured by straight leg raise) without the need for separate hamstring stretching. Looking at a group of soccer players, Castellote-Caballero et al., (2013) used straight leg sliding for three periods over 1 week. Each exercise was practised for 60 seconds for 5 repetitions. Average scores for straight leg raise testing for the control group (no sliding) went from 58.9 degrees to 59.1 degrees, while the intervention group (neural sliding) went from 58.1 degrees to 67.4 degrees.

Exercise **140** Unsupported slump

Starting position and instructions

Sit on a stool with your feet together and unsupported. Link your hands behind you and gently flex your spine, beginning with your neck, to take your chin down to your chest. Continue the movement, rolling through the spine rather than leaning forwards. At the same time, straighten both legs, locking your knees and pulling your feet towards you. Maintain the full stretch for 30 seconds, then slowly release.

Variations

Components of this movement can be used individually at first and then built up into the full sequence. Begin by flexing your trunk and linking your hands behind you. Next, remain upright initially and straighten both knees, pulling your feet towards you. Once both movements can be performed with no pain/tingling, combine the two into a single action.

Points to note

This action stretches the whole of the nervous system, affecting the spinal cord, upper limb nerves and lower limb nerves of both legs. As soon as you feel any tingling or resistance to the stretch, release the movement by flexing your legs slightly and releasing the neck flexion. Maintain this new position for 20–30 seconds and then release. For the next repetition, again go just short of the point of pain/tingling, hoping to push this point further away, enabling you to straighten your legs further while maintaining your trunk flexion.

Exercise **141** Slump – long sitting

Starting position and instructions

The exercise is best performed close to a wall, with the feet pressed against the wall to dorsiflex them. Keeping your legs locked out straight, place your hands by your sides and gradually flex your spine, beginning with the chin to the chest and rolling through the spine, aiming your head towards your hips rather than your knees.

Variations

You can use a yoga belt placed below the balls of your feet instead of the wall. Grip the belt and pull lightly, encouraging your trunk into thoracic flexion and your feet into dorsiflexion.

Perform a long sitting slump slider by bending your knee and spine and then straightening your knee and spine and looking upwards, in a continuous action.

Points to note

Normally, good exercise practice would dictate that spinal alignment be maintained and excessive thoracic flexion avoided. However, the long sitting slump is designed to increase the emphasis on the thoracic spine, and so controlled thoracic flexion is actively encouraged in this movement.

The slump stretch has been shown to be effective in the management of low back pain (Cleland et al., 2006). Choosing low back pain patients with mild symptoms, subjects were assessed using self-report pain measures and a disability index questionnaire (Oswestry Disability Index or ODI). They completed a slump stretch programme, sitting with their legs straight, ankles dorsiflexed (0 degrees) and feet flat against a wall. Overpressure was applied to the cervical spine by a therapist to the point at which the subject's symptoms were produced (fig 13.4a). The position was held for 30 seconds, and 5 repetitions were performed over a period of 3–4 minutes. Patients performed a slump stretch using self-applied overpressure (hands behind head) as home exercise (fig 13.4b). At the end of the study, those who had practised the slump stretch demonstrated a statistically significant improvement of disability score, pain reduction and symptom centralisation.

Figure 13.4 Slump stretch for low back pain

Definition:

Centralisation is a phenomenon seen during the recovery of low back pain with referred pain, normally into the leg. Those with severe conditions may have pain referring through the whole leg and into the foot. As the symptoms subside, they appear further up the leg to the calf or knee, and eventually centralise into the buttock and finally back into the spine.

Exercise 142 Rollover

Exercise 143 Straight leg raise – neural emphasis

Starting position and instructions

The rollover is the classic yoga position called the Plough (Halasana). Lie on the floor on your back and bring your bent legs up over your head, leaving your arms on the floor. Pull your feet towards you (dorsiflexion) and gradually straighten your legs, trying to place your toes on the floor to take some of your bodyweight.

Variations

If you are unable to place your toes on the floor, rest your feet on one or two cushions. With your arms wide, the surface area of support (footprint) is greater. Gripping the hands together reduces the surface area of support, but increases the effect of the stretch to the arms.

Points to note

The rollover has a similar effect to the long sitting slump, but places greater pressure on the thoracic spine and further forces the stretch. This is a specialised neural stretch that is contraindicated in a general exercise programme. If you have a history of lower back pain, you should only attempt it after consulting a physiotherapist.

Starting position and instructions

Lie on the floor on your back and flex one hip, slowly raising the straight leg. At the same time, pull your toes towards you (dorsiflexion). Maintain the full stretch position for 20–30 seconds, then slowly lower.

Variations

The neural component of this stretch is increased by dorsiflexing the foot further, adducting the straight leg and flexing the neck to 'wind-up' the spinal cord from above.

Points to note

The straight leg raising (SLR) movement is used as a test when a person has back pain. The aim is to see if the action produces pain from the back into the buttock and down the leg into the foot. If this is the case, it follows that the sciatic nerve is trapped; this is caused frequently by an intervertebral disc that has bulged or burst into the path of the nerve root at its junction with the spinal cord. The SLR action is a good illustration of the various stages of nerve movement that occur as a stretching exercise is performed. As the leg is raised initially, the sciatic nerve slides through a notch in the pelvis; as the leg is raised further, between 20–30 degrees of hip flexion, the nerve roots start to move past the individual vertebrae. Movement of the nerve past neighbouring structures stops altogether as the leg is raised past 70 degrees. From this position to the full range stretch of 90 degrees, the nerve is stretched like an elastic band. Sliding of the nerve, therefore, occurs below 70 degrees, with stretching only coming on from this range to the end of the straight leg raise movement (*see* fig 13.5).

Figure 13.5 Effects of straight leg raising (SLR):
(a) movement of sciatic nerve begins at the pelvis;
(b) movement of roots begins at the spine;
(c) minimal movement only, but increase in tension

Exercise 144 Active knee extension – neural emphasis

Starting position and instructions
Lie on the floor on your back, flex one of your hips and knees and place your hands behind your knee. Straighten your leg, keeping your knee directly above your hip.

Variations
Greater stress is placed on the nerve, rather than the hamstring muscles, by medially rotating your hip and pulling your foot towards your body (dorsiflexion).

Points to note
Make sure that your knee stays directly above your hip. There is a tendency with this movement to allow your knee to drop downwards so that your leg can be locked. However, the downward movement of the knee actually releases the stretch by reducing hip flexion.

Exercise **145** Straight leg raise – using a doorway – neural emphasis

Starting position and instructions

Lie in a doorway with one leg straight along the floor and the other positioned with the heel on the doorframe. Gradually straighten the wall-supported leg by sliding your heel upwards, keeping it in contact with the doorframe. At the same time, dorsiflex your foot and place overpressure from the hand on to the knee to encourage the last few degrees of movement. The full stretch should be held for 30 seconds.

Variations

As a progression, both legs can be stretched at once by placing them both on the wall.

Points to note

If your heel is allowed to leave the wall support, the stress placed on your spine can be considerable as the low back may be forced into an extension equivalent to a bilateral straight leg raise. At all times, keep your heel in contact with the doorframe or wall.

Exercise **146** Femoral nerve stretch

Starting position and instructions

Standing, flex one of your knees and pull your hip back into extension. At the same time, flex your trunk (spine) and bring your chin down on to your chest (cervical flexion).

Variations

This movement can also be performed lying on your side, in which case the upper leg is the one that is stretched.

Points to note

This is a variation of the rectus femoris stretch (see exercise 6, page 107). In that stretch, the trunk is kept upright to emphasise the effect on the muscle. In the femoral nerve stretch however, the nerve is emphasised by flexing the trunk and cervical spine.

Exercise 147 Branchial nerve stretch

Starting position and instructions

This movement is the same as exercise 81 (*see* page 147), but when performed in the presence of neural tightness it is the nerve rather than the muscles which takes the predominant stretch. Stand side-on to a wall and place your hand on the wall at shoulder height, with your fingers horizontal and facing backwards. Slowly turn your body and head away from the wall, straightening your arm as you do so.

Variations

Pressing down on the stretched shoulder (depression) with the other hand will increase the stretch further.

Points to note

In the arm, three nerves need to be stretched: the radial nerve, the medial nerve and the ulnar nerve. Since all three come from the spinal cord in the thoracic region, they form a meshwork of nerve roots called the brachial plexus. The nerves of the brachial plexus are often stretched by a physiotherapist using the upper limb tension test (ULTT) in the same way that the SLR is used to stretch the lower limb nerves.

Exercise 148 Median nerve stretch

Starting position and instructions

Begin standing and, keeping your shoulder down, adduct your right arm and rotate it outwards. Extend your wrist and supinate your forearm. Take hold of your wrist with your other hand and press your wrist into further extension.

Variations

The stretch can be increased by flexing your neck (looking downwards). Shrugging your shoulders (scapular elevation) reduces the stretch.

Points to note

This exercise stretches the wrist flexors on the front of the forearm. To increase the emphasis on the nerve itself, the cervical flexion is important.

Exercise **149** Radial nerve stretch

Starting position and instructions

Begin standing and keeping your shoulder down, adduct your right arm, rotating it inwards to place it behind the small of your back. Flex your wrist and pronate your forearm. Take hold of your wrist with your other hand and press your wrist into further flexion.

Variations

The stretch can be increased by flexing your neck (looking downwards). Shrugging your shoulders (scapular elevation) reduces the stretch.

Points to note

This exercise stretches the wrist extensors on the back of the forearm. To increase the emphasis on the nerve itself, the cervical flexion is important. This action tensions the radial nerve, for radial nerve sliding see below.

Exercise **150** Radial nerve slider

Starting position and instructions

Begin sitting on a stool or gym bench. Bend your right arm at the elbow and turn your forearm upwards (supination). At the same time tilt your head to the left, away from your arm (cervical lateral flexion). Using a single smooth action, straighten your arm and turn it inward (medial rotation of the shoulder) bending your wrist and fingers to bring the palm upwards. At the same time turn your head to look at your hand combining a twisting and tipping action of your neck (cervical lateral flexion and rotation).

Variations

Divide the action into two separate components, combining them when both are symptom- (pain- or pins and needles-) free. Hold your head still and just move your arm, and then hold your arm still and just move your head.

Points to note

This action slides the radial nerve but maintains its overall length. As your arm straightens the radial nerve is lengthened in the arm, but as the head looks towards the arm the nerve is shortened in the neck.

Exercise 151 Medial nerve slider

Exercise 152 Ulnar nerve stretch

Starting position and instructions

Begin sitting on a stool or gym bench. Bend your right arm at the elbow and turn your forearm upwards (supination). At the same time tilt your head to the left, away from your arm (cervical lateral flexion). Using a single smooth action, straighten your arm and turn it outwards (lateral rotation of the shoulder) opening your hand and stretching your wrist backwards (wrist extension). At the same time turn your head to look at your hand combining a twisting and tipping action of your neck (cervical lateral flexion and rotation).

Variations

Divide the action into two separate components, combining them when both are symptom- (pain- or pins and needles-) free. Hold your head still and just move your arm, and then hold your arm still and just move your head.

Points to note

This action slides the median nerve but maintains its overall length.

Starting position and instructions

Begin sitting and, keeping your shoulder down, abduct your right arm and flex it at the elbow to reach your hand to the side of your head, as though placing the flat of your hand over your ear.

Variations

The stretch can be increased by flexing your neck sideways away from your stretched arm.

Points to note

If the ulnar nerve is very tight, pins and needles will be felt on the outside of the elbow over the 'funny bone'.

Exercise 153 Ulnar nerve slider

Starting position and instructions

Begin sitting on a stool or gym bench. Straighten your right arm and tilt your head to the left. Using a single smooth action, bend your arm and raise it to bring your palm to the side of your head. At the same time tip your head to the right (cervical side flexion) to touch the side of your head to your palm.

Variations

Divide the action into two separate components, combining them when both are symptom- (pain- or pins and needles-) free. Hold your head still and just move your arm, and then hold your arm still and just move your head.

Points to note

This action slides the ulnar nerve but maintains its overall length, reducing nerve tension and increasing nerve motility.

SUMMARY

- There are two types of nerve cell: those that carry electrical impulses and those that protect and support the nerves.
- All the nerves and the spinal cord are linked into a 'continuous tissue tract'.
- Nerves will slide as a limb is stretched.
- After injury, sticky swelling will 'tether' a nerve, reducing its normal movement.
- A nerve has several vulnerable areas where it may be trapped or its movement restricted.
- When a nerve is stretched, its blood flow is reduced. Repeated nerve stretches should therefore be avoided.
- Nerve stretching exercises resemble muscle stretches, but with subtle changes. They must be exact.
- When stretching a nerve, hold the stretch position at a point just short of that at which tingling or pain are felt.

STRETCHING THE FASCIA

14

The concept of working on fascia has a long history in the physical therapies. It was first discussed in the work of Ida Rolf in America, who described a type of bodywork she called 'structural integration'. Most recently, this work has been championed by Tom Myers, Leon Chaitow and Judith DeLany. Myers has produced an excellent book in which he maps the myofascial meridians, and has a number of videos dealing with this subject under the name 'Anatomy Chains'. Chaitow and DeLany have produced two in-depth textbooks dealing with fascial treatment, or 'neuromuscular technique' (NMT). The increasing volume of research on fascia led to the launch of the Fascia Research Congresses and the publication of material by the major contributors in a review book (Schleip et al., 2012). Much of the information for this chapter is taken from these publications, and the reader is referred to them for a more detailed study of this subject. All are listed in the references at the end of the book.

WHAT IS FASCIA?

The body is composed of four basic types of tissue: epithelial, connective, muscular and nervous (*see* table 2.1, page 23). Epithelial tissue covers surfaces or forms structures; for example, it makes up the glands and digestive system. Connective tissue consists of disparate cells floating within an extracellular matrix; depending on the cells present, connective tissue may form cartilage, bone or fascia. Muscular tissue contracts; it forms the muscles we train in the gym, as well as the muscles of the heart and those controlling the hair follicles in the skin. Nervous tissue makes up our nerves, spinal cord and brain.

To find out more about fascia, we need to focus on the connective tissue. Connective tissue is made up of fat (storage) and fibrous tissue (structure). The fibrous tissue contains collagen (white), a strong tough substance that gives the tissue its strength, and elastin (yellow), which gives the tissue its spring. Depending on the concentration of collagen and elastin, the connective tissue is either tough or pliable. Tendons, ligaments and the membranes covering bones and certain portions of the fascia contain mainly white fibres, whereas specific fascia such as the ligamentum flavum in the neck and the wall of blood vessels are mainly yellow elastic tissue.

So, fascia is a type of connective tissue. It links parts of the body together and transmits some of the force created by the muscles. More importantly, it provides a continuous tract covering several bones and muscles leading to a 'line of pull' that is not restricted to a single muscle.

When we study anatomy, we can use imaging such as X-ray or MRI and gross dissection. These techniques have up to now given us a fairly limited knowledge of the complexities of fascia. With dissection, it is possible to separate individual tissues to name and identify them. So, for example we can separate and see the biceps tendon, or the vertebral disc. With fascia, however, this is not practical as fascia is a type of tissue and so more accurately forms a continuous body-wide tension network. Recent developments in high-resolution ultrasound and in-the-body (in vivo) measurement of fascia have revealed a highly complex structure.

TYPES OF FASCIA

Fascia itself is subdivided into two types: superficial and deep. The superficial fascia lies just beneath the skin, acting as a base to enable the skin to move freely over the underlying tissues. A loosely arranged, folded meshwork with the folds filled with fat, the superficial fascia dictates the body contours and gives each of us our unique look. This portion of the fascia is the main place where fat is deposited in obesity, hence the use of skin-fold measurements to assess body-fat percentage.

The fat within the superficial fascia provides us with insulation and is very important in preventing heat loss, especially as we are smooth-skinned rather than furry like a cat. Interestingly, in most other mammals (i.e. those with fur), the superficial fascia does not contain fat. For this reason, the skin of a cat is only loosely connected to the underlying tissue, which is why you can pick the animal up by the scruff of its neck. This is not the case with a person; the skin is too tight! On its under-surface, the superficial fascia becomes more fibrous and forms a distinct layer, which normally then connects to the deep fascia.

The deep fascia is tougher and more fibrous than the superficial fascia and surrounds almost every structure in the body. The deep fascia tends to be laid down in the direction of stress and attaches itself to bony projections as it passes over them. The under-surface of the deep fascia travels between muscle layers as the intermuscular septa, separating the groups of muscles from each other. The muscles are thus grouped in 'compartments' (*see* fig 14.1). In the case of the arms, these are the flexor and extensor compartments, and in the thigh they are the flexor, extensor and adductor compartments, for example.

The fascial membrane takes on a variety of names depending on its anatomical position. Around the brain and spinal cord it is the meninges, around the heart it is the pericardium, within the abdomen it is called the peritoneum and around the bones, it is known as the periosteal. Even within the musculoskeletal system fascia may be specialised. At the side of the leg we have the ilio-tibial band (ITB) and in the back the thoraco-lumbar fascia (TLF). The important feature, however, is that all of the layers of fascia are connected to each other. Fascia is really a 'soft tissue skeleton', as it supports the body, forms boundaries and moulds the shape of the

Figure 14.1 A gross muscle fascia

body tissues. It is not really possible to perform a stretching exercise and affect only one muscle; when we stretch, one muscle may receive the greater stretching effect, but both the muscle and the fascia will change tension. For this reason, we can talk of muscle and fascia as a single inseparable unit called myofascia.

Fascia varies in both density and regularity. Deep fascia is more dense, while superficial fascia is generally loose. Defined structures such as tendons and ligaments have a more regular make-up while fascia proper is largely irregular. Table 14.1 lists named elements of the fascial network.

TRAINING THE FASCIA

We have seen that tissue overload is central to training. Fascia must be overloaded and in so doing demonstrates great adaptability, remodelling effectively through fibroblast activity. Whereas muscle strength increases relatively quickly (*see* Norris, Christopher M., *The Complete Guide to Exercise Therapy* (Bloomsbury, 2013, chapter 3) fascial adaptation is more long-term with 30 per cent of collagen fibres replaced within 6 months and 75 per cent within 24 months (Schleip and Muller, 2013). One of the traditional images of a fascial component in the human body is the muscle-tendon unit (MTU). In the past it was always taught that a muscle contracted to create force and a tendon applied the force but did not create it. Elements of this model are certainly true,

Table 14.1	Elements of the fascial web
Dense connective tissue	Periosteum
Non-dense areolar tissue	Neurovascular tract
Superficial fascia	Epimysium
Intermuscular septa	Perimysium
Interosseous membrane	Endomysium

(Data from Schleip et al., 2012)

in that muscle contracts to create force and tendon does not. However, muscle ultrastructure shows us that fascia occurs in parallel with the muscle as tendon, and in series with the muscle as the muscle framework (epimysium, perimysium). We have seen in chapter 2 that fascia is elastic and can create force (elastic strength) through recoil. The recoil combines with muscle contraction to create both active and passive force, through the *stretch shortening cycle* (SSC). When training performance athletes, SSC consists of an eccentric action (controlled lengthening) immediately followed by a rapid concentric action.

In order to apply stretching to fascia optimally, we must recognise the SSC and apply both static stretching and oscillatory (dynamic) actions. In this chapter we will look at specific static stretches for fascia, while dynamic stretching involving fascia as part of SSC is covered in chapter 11.

Maintaining the elasticity of fascia is one of the most important aims of stretching. It has been shown that fascia is more elastic in the young

Definition:

Fascia is our 'soft tissue skeleton', forming a continuous body-wide tension network.

Key point:

Muscle can create force actively through contraction and passively through recoil of its fascial components.

due to its two-dimensional lattice structure, an architecture which changes to a more haphazard multidirectional alignment with age (Schleip and Muller, 2012). Lack of movement results in a loss of fascial tissue elasticity and reduced tissue gliding. Eventually non-use causes adhesions and fibre matting (Jarvinen et al., 2002).

In addition to alteration in fibre direction, reduced fascia tissue usage can change tissue hydration. Fascia is 70 per cent water in volume, and mechanical loading squeezes the water from the fascia, a little like pressing a sponge. Release of the tension causes rehydration and refreshment of the tissue fluid, so training should be repeated and rhythmical rather than high load and reduced volume.

Also of interest in fascial training is the concept of proprioception. Proprioceptive receptors are located in several structures including joint tissues, muscle and fascia. It is known that proprioception may be impaired through both injury and lack of use, and that exercise is key to its enhancement. However, proprioceptors located within joint structures have been shown to be stimulated at end-range motion and those in fascia more within mid-range, so fascial proprioception may be more important for functional day-to-day activity. Static stretching does overload the proprioceptive system, but focuses on range of motion (movement quantity). Dynamic stretching, especially that involving more complex motion in several planes, is more challenging. In addition, focusing on refining a complex action (movement quality) requires a greater amount of motor skill, demanding more input from the proprioceptive system.

Fascial stretching then, is ultimately dynamic with rhythmic changes in direction using an interplay between muscle contraction and connective tissue elasticity. At the end of an action

Key point:

Focusing on movement quality rather than movement quantity is more demanding to the proprioceptive system.

movement slows down as tissue is stretched and speeds up as the tissue recoils followed by muscle contraction to create active force (ballistic muscle action, *see* chapter 2).

FASCIAL PATHWAYS

According to Myers (2001), there are four main fascial pathways (*see* table 14.2). The superficial back line (SBL) supports the body in full extension, preventing it from collapsing into flexion. It is therefore important in forward bending and lifting tasks. The superficial front line (SFL) transmits muscle force to create powerful flexion of the legs and trunk. The lateral line (LL) is important for single leg actions during walking and running, as well as for lateral bending activities of the trunk. Finally, the spiral line (SL) creates rotational movements of the body, which are important during functional activities such as walking and running, as well as during sport.

Each of the four major fascial pathways links a variety of myofascial structures, which are detailed in table 14.3. When performing any stretch, we can increase the emphasis on the fascial pathways by involving more of these structures. For example, when performing a sit and reach stretch (exercises 26, page 118, and 98, page 159), the stretch works the hamstrings and spine. The myofascial effect on the superficial back line can be increased by bending the spine, touching the chin to the chest and drawing the foot into dorsiflexion.

Table 14.2	Fascial pathways
Pathway	**Position**
Superficial back line	Connects posterior surface of body from toes to knees and then knees to brow.
Superficial front line	Anterior body surface from top of feet to the sides of the skull.
Lateral line	Foot and outside of ankle along the lateral aspect of the leg and trunk to the ear.
Spiral line (takes portions from the other three)	From one side of the skull, across the back to the opposite shoulder and then back across the chest and down the side of the body. From the foot up the back to rejoin the skull fascia.

Table 14.3	Fascial pathways in detail
Superficial back line	• Scalp • Erector spinae and thoroco lumbar fascia • Sacrotuberous ligament • Hamstrings • Gastrocnemius and Achilles • Plantar fascia • Short toe extensors
Superficial front line	• Scalp • Sternomastoid • Sternal fascia • Rectus abdominis • Rectus femoris and quadriceps • Patellar tendon • Toe and foot extensors
Lateral line	• Sternomastoid and deep neck muscles • Intercostals • Lateral abdominals • Gluteus maximus • Tensor fascia lata • Hip abductors • Fibular ligament • Peroneal muscles
Spiral line	• Deep neck muscles (splenius) • Rhomboids • Serratus anterior • Oblique abdominals • Abdominal fascia • Ilio-tibial tract (ITB) • Tibialis anterior • Peroneal longus • Biceps femoris • Sacrotuberous ligament • Erector spinae and thoroco-lumbar fascia

THE SUPERFICIAL BACK LINE (SBL)

Exercise 154 Forward bend – with a belt

Starting position and instructions

Sit on a mat with your legs straight. Bend forwards from the waist, flexing the whole of your trunk and neck, and try to touch your chin to the top of your breastbone. At the same time, pull your feet and toes towards you (dorsiflexion of the ankle and extension of the toes).

Variations

To increase the intensity of the stretch, place a yoga belt or hand towel around your feet and toes and gently pull the toes towards you.

Points to note

This stretch targets the whole of the SBL, involving the plantar fascia, calf and hamstrings, then right up through the spine to the scalp. However, with overpressure from the yoga belt or hand towel, the pressure within the lumbar discs will be increased. This is not recommended for individuals with a history of a disc lesion (slipped disc), unless supervised by a physiotherapist.

Exercise 155 Downward dog

Starting position and instructions

Stand with your feet hip width apart. Keeping your back straight, bend your knees and reach down to touch the floor with your flat hands. Keeping the hands in place, walk your feet backwards until they are 1–1.5 m away from your hands and your body forms an upside down 'V'. Keep your arms straight and press your chest downwards to straighten your back.

Variations

Taking your feet further backwards will bring your legs closer to the horizontal and increase the angle of dorsiflexion at the ankle, placing a greater stretch on the calf and Achilles. Bringing the feet closer to the head will releases some of the stretch on the calf and enable you to press your chest further down, increasing the stretch on the chest and shoulders.

Points to note

This is a classic yoga posture that stretches the SBL while taking some of the flexion stress away from the spine. If you find your feet slipping, practise the position with your heels against a wall. If you are unable to reach the floor, place your hands on a low bench (step bench) instead.

SUPERFICIAL FRONT LINE (SFL)

Exercise 156 Passive full spine extension – with knee flexion

Starting position and instructions

Lie on a mat with your hands beneath your shoulders. Press down with your hands and straighten your arms, arching your back. When you get to the top of the movement, look up towards the ceiling (cervical extension) and bend your knees (knee flexion).

Variations

If you are unable to straighten your arms, place your arms further forwards (a forearm's length in front of the shoulder line) and slightly wider apart (1½ times wider than your shoulders).

Points to note

This exercise, like exercise 80, page 146 forces the lower back (lumbar region) into extension. Encouraging extension in the lumbar region is usually a good thing, unless you have a hollow back (lordotic posture). If this is the case, this movement may be painful, so stop if you feel pain rather than simply tightness in the lower back and seek advice from a physiotherapist or qualified personal trainer.

Exercise 157 Lying overhead reach – with knee flexion

Starting position and instructions

Lie on a gym bench or bed with your bottom supported but your lower thighs off the bed. Bend your knees and at the same time reach overhead, trying to touch the bench above you.

Variations

The SFL stretch can be increased by placing the shoulders on a cushion so that the neck can lower into extension. In addition, pointing the toes and feet (plantarflexion and toe flexion) will target the toe and foot extensors, which form the lower part of the SFL.

Points to note

If you find it too difficult to stretch your arms overhead to touch the bench, place a pillow on the bench above your head and lower your arms on to that instead.

LATERAL LINE (LL)

Exercise 158 Side lying side flexion

Starting position and instructions

Lie on your right side with a pad or folded towel beneath your lower hip if needed (greater trochanter). Place your right hand beneath your right shoulder and press down, stretching your spine into lateral flexion. At the same time, reach your left arm along the outside of your left leg. When your trunk is upright, flex your neck to the left and take a deep breath to expand your ribcage.

Variations

If you are unable to lock your arm out straight, move it further away from your body.

Points to note

As with all side stretches, it is common to find that one side of your body is stiffer than the other. Work on the stiffer side, aiming to regain symmetry rather than increase the range of motion.

Exercise 159 Supported side flexion – with hip adduction

Starting position and instructions

Stand left-side-on to a table or high gym bench and place your left hand on the bench for support. Draw your right leg across and behind your left leg (hip adduction) and reach your right hand overhead, towards your right ear. Bend to the left, taking your bodyweight through your left hand on to the tabletop, and move your left ear towards your left shoulder. Reverse the movement by bending to the right.

Variations

Although the complete movement stretches the whole of the LL, you can add the components gradually. First, perform the hip adduction with trunk side flexion. Second, perform the overhead reach and neck side flexion. When you are comfortable with both movements, combine the two into a single action as described above.

Points to note

It is common to have an asymmetrical body, so do not be surprised if one side of your body is stiffer than the other. Work on the stiffer side, aiming to regain symmetry rather than simply to increase the range of motion.

SPIRAL LINE

Exercise 160 Lying spinal rotation – with leg straightening

Exercise 161 Prone lying leg adduction – with lateral flexion and rotation

Starting position and instructions

Lie on the floor with your left leg bent and right leg straight. Tuck your right hip beneath you and twist your spine to the right, lowering your left knee to the floor. Gradually straighten your left leg and take hold of your shin or foot with your right hand. Keep your left arm on the ground straight out to the side and look to the left. Reverse the movement to target the right side.

Variations

If you find it difficult to hold your shin or foot, wrap a yoga belt or small towel around your shin or foot and hold that instead.

Points to note

As you perform this exercise you will often note a 'click' or 'pop' from the spine. This is normally the release of gas bubbles within the small facet joints of the spine and is harmless. If the click is painful, however, stop the exercise and rest. If the pain continues, consult a physiotherapist.

Starting position and instructions

Lie on your front with your arms out to your sides, bent at the elbow. Your chest and head should be flat on the floor. Lift your right leg and take it across your left (adduction). As you do this, allow your trunk to flex to the left and rotate slightly, opening the right side of your ribcage. Reverse the movement to focus on the left side of the body.

Variations

This movement may be combined with spinal extension (see exercise 156, page 207) to stretch the abdominal fascia as well as the oblique abdominals. To do this, place the hands under the shoulders and press into the ground to extend the spine, then come up on to the elbows or flat hands.

Points to note

If you have limited hip flexibility this movement may not be suitable. Where the hip does not extend easily, the lumbar spine tends to extend too much instead (hyperextension).

PART **THREE**

PRACTICAL APPLICATION

15

Trigger points (TrP) are highly sensitive focal areas within a tight muscle. They are often painful at rest, and can refer pain through an area, causing it to spread away from the TrP along a limb, for example. Take a TrP in the supraspinatus muscle at the top of the shoulder blade. This may be painful if someone digs their fingers into the area, and the pain may spread out across the upper back and even down into the arm. In severe cases, where the TrP is very active, pain may travel down the arm right into the fingers.

A TrP can be one of two types. One that is painful nearly all the time, and the client is aware of, is called an active TrP. Sometimes, however, a client may have pain in an area that has been referred from a TrP, which they were not aware of. In this case the TrP is said to be latent. In the case of the supraspinatus example above, the client may have been aware of arm pain but not the TrP at the top of the shoulder blade. In this case the supraspinatus TrP is latent.

Definition:

An active trigger point is one of which a client is aware. A latent TrP is one where the client is aware of general pain in another body area, made worse by pressing the TrP.

TRIGGER POINT DEVELOPMENT

A number of factors can lead to the development of a TrP (*see* table 15.1).

Psychological factors typically include anxiety and stress, and lead to TrP development in the so-called 'emotional muscles'. These include the neck and shoulders, and lower back. Prolonged stress may lead to TrP development especially in the upper trapezius, and erector spinae. Biomechanical factors include posture. Sitting at a computer, slouched forwards, allows the scapulae to move outwards (scapular abduction) overstretching the rhomboid muscles.

This gives rise to rhomboid TrPs with local pain along the inner edge of the scapula. Muscle injury as a result of overuse or trauma can lead

Table 15.1	Important factors in trigger point development	
Psychological	**Biomechanical**	**Chemical**
Depression	Posture	Toxic chemicals
Anxiety	Trauma (sudden injury)	Nutrient deficiency
Stress	Overuse (gradual injury)	Allergic reaction
Fear		

to TrP development, often giving secondary pain once the original injury has resolved. An example here would be a simple sprained ankle, which damages the lateral ligament on the outside of the ankle. Initially pain and swelling occur at the ankle, but the peronei muscles along the outside of the shin will work hard to protect the ankle. The result can be a peroneus TrP some months after the original injury has resolved. Pain gives 'lateral shin splints' creating tightness over the outer shin after prolonged walking or running.

Interestingly, there are several biochemical factors that have been linked to TrP development. These include reactions to allergens and deficiencies in certain vitamins, especially the B vitamins. It is likely that these factors, while not actually causing individual TrPs, could make a person more susceptible to them. If a client is developing TrPs repeatedly in different muscles they should seek advice from their GP.

PHYSIOLOGY

Trigger points commonly begin when one of the muscle membranes is damaged either by repeated movements (overuse) or a sudden mis-timed pull (trauma). The membrane damage alters the release of the chemical acetylcholine, which is involved in muscle contraction. This chemical is a neurotransmitter (nerve impulse chemical) which spreads across the muscle causing contraction when a nerve impulse arrives from the brain and spinal cord. The change in acetylcholine release causes a parallel alteration in calcium levels at the junction (synapse) between the end of the nerve and the muscle – the so-called 'neuromuscular junction'. Muscle contraction occurs because of this chemical imbalance, and the contraction simply continues even though no nervous impulses are being sent out. When a muscle contracts normally, nerve impulses travel to the muscle and the resulting electrical impulses can be measured on an EMG machine. The stronger the contraction, the greater the signal (amplitude) of the EMG, but where a TrP exists, electrical activity is detected in the muscle even when no nervous impulses are present. This feature, called spontaneous electrical activity (SEA), is a measure which can be used in hospitals to identify a TrP and know when it has been successfully treated.

Key point:

Both chemical and electrical changes occur in a muscle which develops a trigger point.

The permanent contraction of a few local muscle fibres gives a nodule, which is often felt when pressing into a TrP. The contraction restricts local blood flow allowing poisons to accumulate in the area, giving a burning pain, typical of TrPs.

Because the nodule causes local contraction of a few muscle fibres, the bunching pulls on the muscle causing the second feature often seen with TrPs, a taut band. This appears like a cord within the muscle which you can flick your fingers over, and is a familiar feature to massage therapists.

Although TrPs are obviously painful, that is not their only feature. The chemical and mechanical changes which occur also cause the muscle to

Key point:

The two key features of a trigger point are a nodule within the muscle and a taut band.

weaken, allowing further posture changes. Getting rid of the TrP is therefore a primary aim, in the short term it will relieve pain, but in the long term by allowing postural correction it can prevent further problems.

IDENTIFYING A TRIGGER POINT

If you have a TrP yourself, you can usually feel it by pressing your fingers into the painful area. But, how can you identify a TrP in a client? Well, the tightening of the TrP restricts impulses conducted through local nerves. A nerve has a feeling (sensory) function giving pain, and a movement (motor) function giving muscle-weakness. However, the third characteristic of the nerve comes from its sympathetic nerve fibres. These control a number of features including skin condition. As a result subtle skin changes can be seen in the region of a long-lasting TrP, especially on the back. These include altered regions of sweating making the skin tacky or powdery and dry. Skin puckering known as 'orange peel skin' is often noticeable, and there may be a change in the stretchiness of the skin itself. These characteristic types of skin appearance are known as trophic changes. To be seen they require close inspection and may be more easily identified by gently gliding your fingers over the skin surface.

Key point:

Trophic skin changes, which occur when a TrP has been present for a prolonged period, include dry powdery skin, tacky skin, skin puckering and loss of elasticity.

RELEASE TECHNIQUES

There is a number of techniques which we can use to get rid of a TrP and allow the muscle to stretch normally. These are used before stretching, or as part of a gentle stretching action. Once the TrP is released, the muscle must be slowly stretched to its optimal level, comparing it to the unaffected side of the body.

COMPRESSION

Compression techniques include pressing the areas of the trigger point with a tool such as a ball or foam roller, and ischaemic compression, a local massage technique which you can apply to yourself or your partner. Often termed myofascial release, these techniques use a sustained pressure over a TrP which gradually distorts the tissues. By holding the pressure on for 90–120 seconds, the tissues gradually become more fluid. This is a little like pressing hard on to a piece of putty or plasticine. As you press, you will gradually feel the hardness of the TrP ease off and pain will subside. What is happening here is a reversal of the process which follows the onset of a TrP. We saw that blood flow is reduced as a result of TrP formation. This in turn causes dehydration of the tissues stiffening them. The compression technique causes a temporary tissue dehydration which when released allows water molecules to seep back into the area, and fresh blood to return, effectively flushing the region.

Applying compression

Compression may be applied using the fingers and hands (yours or that of a therapist or training partner), or by using a massage tool such as a ball or foam roller (*see* fig 15.1).

Fingers

Direct compression may be given with the flat of your fingers or your hand. Slide your fingers into

Figure 15.1 Massage tools

Figure 15.2 Applying compression with fingers

the tissues along the muscle length. Initially, use a gentle pressure across the surface of the skin like massage. As tension eases, increase the pressure as though you were trying to actually stretch the skin. Finally, maintain the pressure over the TrP and apply a gentle stretch to the underlying muscle. If you have very flexible fingers which hyperextend, use two or three fingers pressed together as a single unit to take the stress off your hands (*see* fig 15.2).

Ball and knobbler

When using a ball, there is a combination of compression and skin stimulation depending on the ball surface. A plain ball (tennis ball) has a smooth surface and may be used for direct compression. The firmer the ball the more local the pressure. A slightly flatter, softer ball spreads the pressure over a larger, more diffuse area. A spiky ball has a series of fairly sharp plastic or rubber spines which gently dig into the skin, increasing skin stimulation. A knobbler is a small ball on the end of a stick which is used as a handle to grip the unit. These may be smaller to fit into the hand, or longer to reach areas between your shoulder blades or lower back. The ball on the knobbler end is smaller and firmer than a tennis

ball, giving a smaller area of stimulation to achieve a greater trigger point localisation.

Foam roller

Foam rollers may be used for direct compression or firm local massage. The rollers come in different diameters and with a variety of surfaces. Smaller diameter (10 cm) rollers have a smaller contact area than larger diameter ones (15 cm). Pressure is greater with a smaller diameter roller, and may be further increased using a roller with prominent ridges or projections (*see* fig 15.3). A local massage effect (fascial release) may be achieved by placing the roller on the floor or

Figure 15.3 Foam rollers

against a wall and moving the body or single limb over it. Taking more of the limb weight on to the roller increases direct local pressure, taking more bodyweight on to your hands and off the roller reduces pressure. The limb is moved across the roller for a range of 15–20 cm to apply local massage, and the technique is carried out for 30–120 seconds. The sensation is a deep ache, which should reduce over time. If the technique is very painful or if the deep sensation/pain increases over the time of application, the rolling should be stopped as it is irritating the condition.

POSITIONAL RELEASE

Positional release works not by stretching a tight muscle, but by taking stress off the tissues so that the muscle can 'reset' itself and allow the TrP to release. The thought here is that prolonged occurrence of a TrP causes the body to 'remember' pain and exaggerate it even when the original cause of the pain has long gone. Positional release works by affecting the pain nerves and the positional (proprioceptive) nerves connected to the tissue with the TrP.

Get your client to press on the TrP and feel how painful it is. They should then move the limb around, until they find a position which reduces the pain of the TrP – the so-called 'position of ease'. This new, less painful position is held for 90–120 seconds and then the TrP is reassessed. Because tight muscles often pull joints out of alignment, there may also be TrPs in the muscles opposite to that which is painful, so search these out as well.

PNF STRETCHING

We have covered PNF stretching on page 61. We know that it is a technique which reduces tone in a muscle and so is ideal as a follow up to TrP release. Once the TrP begins to ease, use PNF stretching to normalise the tone in the affected muscle and then emphasise correct alignment in general movements.

TARGETING AFFECTED MUSCLES

Exercise 162 Upper trapezius

Starting position and instructions

Sit upright on a chair or gym bench. Rest your left hand over your right shoulder and tip your head to the left (left lateral flexion of the neck). Grip your three central fingers together into a single unit, and press this into the TrP within your trapezius muscle. Press the area gently while maintaining the stretched position. As the muscle pain subsides, increase the stretch by laterally flexing your neck further.

Variations

Flex or rotate your neck to vary the effect of the stretch. Actively depress the right shoulder blade (pull it downwards) to stabilise the scapula against the ribcage. Use a light massage stroke across the fibres of the muscle, from front to back.

Points to note

As you apply this stretch, make sure you do not flex the thoracic spine, or raise the right shoulder.

Exercise 163 Pec major

Starting position and instructions

Lie on your back on the floor. Move your left arm out to the side. Use your right hand to locate and press the trigger point within the muscle either close to the breastbone (the sternal head of the pec major) or close to the collarbone (the clavicular head). Press the trigger point and stroke slowly along the muscle in a diagonal direction from chest to shoulder. As the trigger point releases, allow the muscle to stretch further.

Variations

If your pec major is quite tight, rest your forearm on a cushion initially to reduce the stretch. As the muscle lengthens, stretch further to the floor. If, on the other hand, you are very flexible and find the floor stretch easy, lie on a gym bench and allow your arm to stretch below the horizontal level.

Points to note

When the pec major is tight you have a round shouldered posture. However, this normally goes with tightness of the upper (thoracic) spine as well, and this can be stretched using exercises page 111.

Exercise **164** Pec minor

Starting position and instructions

Lie on the floor and get your training partner to place a weight bag over the front of your right shoulder so that your shoulder is pressed right on to the floor. Find the ball of your shoulder joint with the fingers of your left hand and move your fingers downwards and inwards towards your feet until you hit the first couple of ribs. This is where you will find the pec minor trigger point. Press on it and maintain the pressure as you allow your shoulder to relax and be pressed further into the floor by the weight bag.

Variations

Lie on your front with your shoulder on a shallow cushion and allow your body weight to press your shoulder backwards.

Points to note

The pec minor muscle lifts your upper ribs when you take a very deep breath. To lengthen the muscle further, breathe out forcefully as you apply the stretch.

Exercise **165** Supraspinatus

Starting position and instructions

Sit on a gym bench with your right hand behind the small of your back. Reach across your shoulder and place your fingers into the muscles at the top/back of your shoulder below the trapezius. Gently press into this area until you find the trigger point and then massage it in a horizontal direction until it releases.

Variations

Use a contract-relax (CR) technique to release the muscle further. Press your forearm into your back (resisted lateral or outward rotation), hold this tension for 10–20 seconds and then release.

Points to note

The supraspinatus may develop two trigger points; one in its muscle belly at the top of the shoulder blade (scapula), the other at its insertion on to the top of the arm bone (humerus). To locate the humeral trigger point press on the front of the shoulder as you perform the stretch described above.

Exercise 166 Splenius capitus

Exercise 167 Quadratus lumborum (QL)

Starting position and instructions

Sit on a chair and place your fingertips on the area of your skull behind your ears. Gently draw your chin inwards as though trying to give yourself a double chin and try to look downwards at the top of your breastbone. By doing this you should lift the back of your head upwards slightly in a rocking action (Pilates skull rock exercise). Gently massage the tender trigger points in the muscle, and as they release pull the chin in further.

Variations

Where one muscle is tighter than the other, tip your head to that side (lateral flexion) and turn your head towards the muscle (rotation). The combination of lateral flexion and rotation will increase the stretch on the muscle.

Points to note

Splenius capitus is a small deep muscle which lies beneath the trapezius and sternomastoid. It travels from the lower neck to a bone behind your ear (mastoid process) and the lower rim of the back of your skull (nuchal line). Its importance lies in the fact that it develops tenderness and can be the cause of headaches if you spend a lot of time on a computer with your chin poking forwards.

Starting position and instructions

Stand side-on to a high bench or table with your left side to the outside. Bend over sideways towards the table and support yourself on your right hand. Draw your left hand up and press your thumb into the muscles between your pelvis and lower ribs, midway between your spine (erector spinae) and the side of your body (obliques). Find the trigger point and compress it for 90–120 seconds. As your muscle releases and the trigger point pain reduces, allow yourself to side bend further.

Variations

You may also perform this exercise side bent over a gym ball, using your upper hand to locate and release the trigger point.

Points to note

To fully stretch the QL, you must move your pelvis and ribcage apart. In standing this can be better achieved by dipping your hip on the tight side so that the pelvis tips down laterally to this side. When taking a deep breath, the QL pulls the lower rib downwards to help fill the lungs fully. To increase the stretch on the muscle, exhale fully to allow the lower rib to move up.

Exercise 168 Rhomboids

Starting position and instructions

Place a tennis ball on the floor and lie on your side so that the ball is level with the middle of your shoulder blades. Place the rhomboids on stretch by gripping your opposite shoulders, right hand to left shoulder and left to right. This 'self hugging' position will draw your shoulder blades apart (scapular abduction) and place the rhomboids on stretch. Roll from your side to your back so that the tennis ball is squashed beneath your back. Shuffle so

that the ball is placed between your spine and the inner edge of your shoulder blade, over the most painful area which is the trigger point. Allow your bodyweight to press you downwards and maintain the position for 90–120 seconds breathing normally (make sure you don't hold your breath).

Variations

You may use a golf ball instead of a tennis ball. This will give a greater pressure as it is harder, but be careful not to rest your spinal bones on the ball.

Points to note

The rhomboid trigger point may form when the muscle is lengthened rather than shortened, in a round shouldered position. This is because the scapulae move apart, and the rhomboid muscles are trying hard to hold the scapulae back, but failing (eccentric muscle action). You are therefore trying to release the trigger point and reduce muscle pain with this exercise, rather than simply lengthen the muscle.

Exercise 169 Erector spinae

Starting position and instructions

Sit on the floor with your knees bent to 90 degrees, your training partner kneeling behind you. Locate a painful trigger point within the bulk of the erector

spinae to the side of the spine. Get your training partner to press into this area using their knuckle or elbow, as you bend (flex) your spine moving your head towards your upper thighs.

Variations

Your training partner may also stand behind you and place their knee into the trigger point. Combine flexing and rotation of your spine, moving your head towards your opposite thigh.

Points to note

When you stretch in this way there is a greater emphasis on the upper portion of the erector spinae. If your trigger point is very low down close to your pelvis, an alternative stretch is to lie on the floor and bring your knees into your chest, lifting your tailbone from the floor (posterior pelvic tilt).

Exercise **170** Piriformis

Starting position and instructions
Lie on the floor and place a tennis ball beneath your right (painful) buttock. Move around until the ball presses into your painful trigger point. Compress the trigger point until the pain subsides, and then draw your leg up, place your right hand on your right knee and hold your right foot with your left hand. Impart the stretch on to piriformis by drawing your foot towards you and pressing your knee away. This action will rotate your hip joint outwards (lateral rotation) while keeping it in a bent (flexed) position.

Variations
Rather than using your hands, you can perform the stretch using the knee of your other leg (*see* gluteal stretch – lying, exercise 2, on page 105).

Points to note
This muscle lies over the sciatic nerve, the major nerve that passes through your buttock and into your thigh. It is common for compression of this area to give tingling (pins and needles) into your leg. If this occurs, release the pressure slightly until the tingling goes away.

Exercise **171** Hamstrings – direct pressure

Starting position and instructions
Stand with your painful leg bent and the heel resting on a low bench or table below waist height. Push your fingers into the trigger point on the back of your thigh. As the pain subsides, gently press your leg straighter by sliding your heel out along the bench.

Variations
A greater stretch is given using a higher bench, and sliding the leg slightly sideways, outwards (hip abduction) or inwards (hip adduction) will change the emphasis of the stretch.

Points to note
The upper portion of the hamstrings will receive a greater stretch using an anterior tilt of the pelvis (tail forwards) rather than a posterior tilt (tipping your tail backwards).

Exercise 172 Hamstrings – on a foam roller

Exercise 173 TFL/ITB

Starting position and instructions

Begin sitting on the floor with your legs straight. Place a 15 cm foam roller beneath your left thigh and put your hands behind you onto the floor. Bend your right leg and take your weight on to your hands and right foot, to lift your body slightly. Lower your bodyweight on to the roller to apply enough pressure to identify the trigger point but not cause pain. Move yourself forward and backwards over the roller in a smooth sweeping action of about 10–15 cm. Perform 8–12 reps and then rest to allow fresh fluid into your tissues.

Variations

Use a smaller (10 cm) roller on one with projections to increase the skin stimulus. Wear a pair of thin trousers (jogging bottoms) to reduce skin stimulation.

Points to note

Usually pain will increase before the trigger point releases and pain reduces. Allowing the knee to bend slightly will take stretch off the hamstrings and allow the trigger point to release more easily.

Starting position and instructions

Lie on your back and bend your painful (right) leg. Cross it over your left leg. Locate your painful trigger point on the side of your thigh and press it until the pain subsides. Stretch the TFL/ITB by using the weight of your top (right) leg to press your bottom (left) leg across your body into adduction.

Variations

Varying the bend at the knee will alter the emphasis of the stretch.

Points to note

The stretch on the ITB/TFL must be maintained for a long period (2–3 minutes) to get the full effect.

Exercise 174 TFL/ITB – using a foam roller

Starting position and instructions
Begin lying on your left side with your legs straight and a foam roller placed beneath your left thigh. Prop yourself up on your hands and bend your right knee to place your foot flat on the ground. Press on to your hands and right foot to take some of your bodyweight and lower yourself on to the roller. Move your body up and down (10–15 cm) pressing the roller into the painful trigger point area. Perform 8–12 repetitions before resting to allow tissue recovery.

Variations
Lie on your right side and keep both legs straight, placing the roller beneath your right thigh. Maintain constant pressure by staying in place for 20–30 seconds.

Points to note
Trigger points to the ITB are frequently located in the lower third of the band, about 10–15 cm above the side of the knee, or in the upper portion around the greater trochanter.

Exercise 175 Anterior shin – using a spiky ball and foam roller

Starting position and instructions
Begin standing with your left leg against a wall. Place a spiky ball or foam roller between the wall and your upper shin, situated at the point of greatest tenderness. Lean into the wall to increase pressure on the ball/roller and move your leg up and down using a hip hitch action.

Variations
This action can also be performed lying on the floor with the ball between your shin and the floor.

Points to note
This movement targets trigger points in the tibialis anterior muscle. This muscle is affected in shin splints (compartment syndrome) where pain is on the front and outside (antero-lateral) aspect of the shin. Other muscles are affected with other forms of shin pain, including the peronei (lateral pain), and deep toe flexors (medial pain). *See* Norris, Christopher M., *Managing Sports Injuries* (Churchill Livingstone, Oxford, 2011), pages 210–215, for more details.

MEASURING
FLEXIBILITY

16

WHY WE NEED TO MEASURE FLEXIBILITY

Flexibility should be measured in order to:
- determine your existing range of motion;
- assess any muscle imbalance;
- chart your progress as you train.

RANGE OF MOTION

When a muscle is more flexible than normal (hyperflexible), there is no need to stretch it, and in fact to do so could leave you open to injury. If a muscle is too flexible, there may not be enough strength in the muscles supporting the joint to control the total range of motion, in such a case, we say that hyperflexibility (greater than normal range of motion) has developed into instability (inability to control joint alignment through the whole available range).

> **Definition:**
>
> Hyperflexibility is simply a greater amount of flexibility than the average person has. Instability is the inability to control and maintain the alignment of a body part, especially the lower back.

MUSCLE IMBALANCE

You will also need to assess the ratio of muscle flexibility on one side of the joint to that on the opposing side. When there is a marked difference in flexibility or strength between the two, muscle imbalance is present (*see* page 42) and it would be wrong to undertake an overall stretching programme. This would simply allow the imbalance to continue although the muscles, in general, would all be more flexible. When an imbalance is detected, the answer is to stretch only those muscles that are too tight, and to strengthen and shorten those that are too loose (flabby) by exercising in the inner-range position. Once the imbalance has been corrected, a general flexibility programme can be used.

CHARTING PROGRESS

Stretching is a long-term part of any training programme, so you will need 'goals' or targets to aim for. In order to do this, you will need to measure your flexibility and aim at improving it within a certain time. For example, you might aim at improving the range of motion of a joint by a certain number of degrees in a certain number of months; or aim to reach far enough to touch a certain point by a set date (for instance, Christmas or birthdays). Either way, the goals you set yourself must be specific and realistic. It is no good simply saying that you want to increase your flexibility, because this is too open-ended: increase it by how much, and in how long? Your goals must also be realistic: you may never be able to perform the splits if you are over 50 and very inflexible in the hip adductors. This really does not matter, provided that your degree of flexibility is appropriate to your age, body make-up and activity level. Remember, the right amount of stretching is the right amount for you as an individual. There is no competition – no winners and no losers. When goals are set, you are only really competing with yourself, so the goals must be acceptable to you.

Key point:

When setting goals, the mnemonic SMART is useful. Your goals should be specific, measurable, acceptable, realistic and timed.

HOW TO MEASURE FLEXIBILITY

USING A SCORE CHART

The flexibility tests, illustrated in table 16.1 (*see* pages 231–235), can be used as a test to measure your flexibility. Average values are quoted, but they are for general guidance only. If you have a specific problem that limits your flexibility, you should see your physiotherapist or personal trainer.

You should perform a warm-up before testing any movement, and wear warm clothing to keep your body warm while performing the tests. Make sure that you perform the same degree of warm-up each time you measure your flexibility. The exercises are either static or active stretches (*see* pages 59 and 60) and should be performed

slowly and held in the stretched position. There should be no bobbing or bouncing actions, which will give a deceptively high score. The instructions for each exercise are included in the table.

CLINICAL FLEXIBILITY TESTING

The score chart can only give a rough, but still very useful, guide to flexibility. Where a more precise measurement is needed, clinical testing is used. This accurately measures the angle of the joint at the point of maximal stretch, and is called goniometry. A number of goniometers are available. The simplest is the universal goniometer (*see* fig 16.2). This consists of a 180-degree or 360-degree protractor. It has a single axis and scale, but two arms. One arm is held stationary, the axis of the goniometer is placed on the axis (centre) of the joint to be measured, and the two arms rest on the mid-lines of the bones on either side of the joint. The joint angle obtained when stretching is read from the centre scale.

The gravity goniometer consists of a needle inside a fluid-filled container. The needle points downwards due to gravity and acts as a reference against which the joint range is measured. The goniometer is strapped on to the limb and a direct reading is achieved.

If you want to measure your flexibility when performing a certain sports action, the simplest way is to take a picture of the action and then to measure the movement on the photograph. This is made easier by drawing lines along the long axis of the bones and then using a simple school protractor to measure the angle between the two lines. Remember however, that the angle of the camera can change the appearance of the limbs and so, to be truly objective, you should really position the camera in the same position each time you take a photograph of a particular action.

1 Shoulder girdle

180°
90°
20–40°
0°

(a) Abduction-
adduction

150–170°
–90°
40°
0°

(b) Elevation-
extension

2 Elbow and forearm joints

130°
10°

(a) Flexion-
extension

0°
80–90°   80–90°

(b) Supination-
pronation

3 Hip joint

130–140°

(a) Flexion

10°

(b) Extension

130°

(c) Flexion

4 Knee joint

5–10°
0°
120–150°

Flexion-extension

5 Ankle joint

20–30°
0°
40–50°

Plantar flexion-dorsal
extension of the ankle joint

30–45°
0°   20–30°

(d) Abduction-adduction
in supine position

30–45°   40–50°
0°

(e) Internal/external rotation
in supine position with
hip joint bent

Figure 16.1 Joint centres and motion range

Figure 16.2 the goniometer

mid-line of lower leg

mid-line of upper leg

axis of joint

(a)

(b)

Figure 16.3 Correct goniometer position: (a) correct alignment of goniometer with arms along mid-line of limb; (b) incorrect alignment gives appearance of reduced range of motion

How to use the goniometer

Figure 16.2 shows the plan for a simple goniometer. Photocopy this, stick the copy on to a piece of firm card or plastic and cut out the shape. Fasten the two pieces together with a clip. The goniometer is now ready for use.

To take a reading, position point A over the centre of rotation of the joint. This is the point of the joint around which the movement appears to take place. Figure 16.1 shows the centres of rotation for the large joints. To maintain accuracy, the arms of the goniometer must be positioned parallel to the bones along the mid-line of the limb. Figures 16.3(a) and 16.3(b) show correct and incorrect alignment respectively. In figure 16.3(b), the upper arm of the goniometer is not aligned along the mid-line of the upper leg, so the reading obtained is lower, giving the appearance of a less flexible joint.

ACCURACY IN MEASUREMENTS

SPINE AND HIP MOVEMENT

When the spine is moving in combination with either the lower limb or upper limb, close examination is required to determine which joints are actually taking part in the stretching exercise. Tightness in the ligaments surrounding the hip means that, once the hip has flexed beyond 90 degrees, the pelvis starts to tilt and the lower spine subsequently begins to flex. Total range of motion may be made up of movements at a number of joints. In figure 16.4(a), the individual appears to have long hamstrings because he is able to touch his toes. In fact, the hamstrings are short and the pelvis has stayed tilted back. The movement is occurring in the lumbar spine because the individual's spinal extensors are excessively flexible. In figure 16.4(b), the range of motion

| (a) | (b) | (c) |

Figure 16.4 Sit-and-reach test – what is being measured? (a) excessive flexibility in spinal extensions; (b) excessive rounding of thoracic spine; (c) normal back flexion and short hamstrings

appears normal, but neither the hamstrings nor the spinal extensors are flexible. Instead the movement is coming from the thoracic spine, which is rounding excessively. In figure 16.4(c), the hamstrings are also short, but like those of the individual in figure 16.4(a), the spinal extensors are of average length, so the total range of motion is considerably reduced.

PELVIC AND HIP MOVEMENT

Pelvic tilt is also an important factor in determining hip motion. In figures 16.5(a) and 16.5(b), the length of the rectus femoris is being measured. In figure 16.5(a), no pelvic tilt is occurring and the range of hip extension is seen to be limited. In figure 16.5(b), the same range of hip extension is occurring, but the anterior tilt of the pelvis, occurring at the same time, gives the appearance of an increase in total range of motion.

SPINE AND SHOULDER MOVEMENT

Movement of the spine with the shoulder is also important. In figures 16.6(a) and 16.6(b), the range of shoulder elevation is being measured against the wall. In figure 16.6(a), the movement is seen to be limited, but in figure 16.6(b) there appears to be a greater range of motion. In fact, the range of motion at the shoulder is exactly the

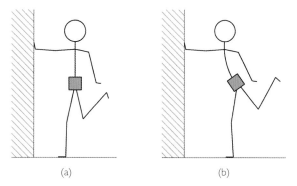

| (a) | (b) |

Figure 16.5 Pelvic tilt and hip extension

same in each case; it is the movement occurring in the spine that is greater in the second figure.

When measuring joint movement, it is essential to limit the motion to a single joint. This can be achieved by looking closely at the body and repeating the movement to ensure accuracy.

USING FLEXIBILITY MEASURES IN RESEARCH STUDIES

When flexibility measures are being used as part of a research study, as discussed in chapter 6, we need to be sure that the tests are both accurate and giving us the information that we think they

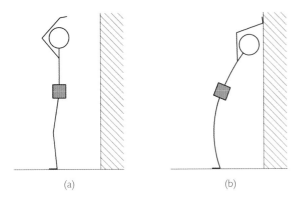

(a)   (b)

Figure 16.6 Spine and shoulder movements

are. Although a full discussion of experimental design and research techniques is not within the scope of this book, we will look at some of the fundamental processes. The interested reader is referred to Thomas and Nelson (1990) for further information.

Validity and reliability are two essential factors in measurement error. Validity asks the question, 'Does the test measure what it claims to do?', whereas reliability asks, 'Was each test of a batch the same?' Both are essential for maintaining the accuracy of stretching tests.

VALIDITY

Take the example of a straight leg raise (SLR) action to measure hamstring length. We perform a certain number of stretches over six weeks and use the SLR to determine the best number of stretches for increasing hamstring flexibility. Is this a valid measure?

Key point:

Validity asks, 'Does the test measure what we think it does?', reliability asks, 'Was each test really the same?'

There are two types of validity: internal and external. Internal validity refers to the extent to which the results of a study can be attributed to the exercises (intervention) used. For example, if flexibility on the SLR does increase after six weeks, was this the result of our stretching programme or something else, such as the passage of time? External validity is concerned with the generalisation of the results. In other words, are the changes that occurred in our experiment likely to occur outside the laboratory situation? Sometimes, an experiment may be so controlled that it no longer reflects what occurs in sport. For example, if we choose to measure the SLR lying flat and using a frame that fixes the pelvis and prevents the knee from bending to ensure accuracy, how does this compare to a football-kicking action where the hamstrings are stretched in sport? Clearly, there may be so many differences that the exercise is no longer the same as the functional action.

Internal validity

A number of factors may affect internal validity:

- History can affect internal validity if some other event occurred at the same time as testing that could have affected the results. For example, if we used students for our experimental subjects, some of them may have started a gymnastic programme at school at the same time as the experiment, and they may well have used hamstring stretching as part of their gymnastics. This makes it impossible to say whether our study, or the gymnastics, was responsible for any results obtained.
- Maturation refers to the passage of time. This is important when a study, especially with children, lasts for a prolonged period. For example, if we have a group of 10-year-olds and our study lasts for two to three years, are any results simply the effect of moving into

adolescence and the flexibility changes that occur during this time?

- Testing will itself affect the results. Once we have measured hamstring length using the SLR, we have in fact stretched the hamstrings with the SLR test. The subjects have learned how to perform the test, and may be able to relax their muscles further.

- Instrumentation changes are also very important. For example, if we are using a goniometer (*see* page 227), the position of the goniometer and the type of goniometer used must remain the same; otherwise, the measurement obtained will be different, not through stretching, but through inaccurate measurement.

- Statistical regression is a tendency for factors to vary, especially if extreme measures (very flexible or very inflexible) are used. If we choose a group with very tight hamstrings for our study, we would expect them to vary in such a way as to move towards the average score. This is because all scores will vary with each measurement; sometimes a person is more flexible, and sometimes less. We are only measuring an average for that individual, and that average will constantly change.

- Selection biases encompass the number of factors involved in picking subjects for the study in the first place. For example, if we ask for volunteers for a flexibility study, we may well get a lot of individuals who think they are flexible (we all like to show off!). Equally, those who stay with the study (six weeks is a long time) are likely to be those who are enjoying it, or have a particular reason to do it (perhaps it is a requirement for their college course).

External validity

When dealing with threats to external validity, remember that we are concerned with whether our results accurately reflect what happens in the real world.

- If we use a pre-test, i.e. we allow an individual to get used to the experimental set-up before we test them, we may get reactive effects of testing. The subject would be prepared for the test and aware of what was coming. This would not occur on the sports field, for example, where the stretch would be performed during an exercise.

- We must also be careful that the way we select individuals for our study does not interact with the measurement we are using. For example, test results from subjects who know where their hamstrings are may differ from subjects who do not have this knowledge.

- If the results of our testing only occur in the laboratory but not in the real world, we are seeing reactive effects of the experimental set-up. For example, we may choose to take a measurement with a very complex piece of apparatus that influences movement to such a degree that the movement is no longer similar to the one used in sport.

- If two or more stretches are given, the effects of one exercise may influence the other, and we have multiple treatment interference.

Key point:

Internal validity asks whether the results of a study are really due to the stretching exercises used (known as the 'intervention'). External validity asks whether the results obtained in a laboratory experiment actually mirror the results that would have occurred in the real world.

Table 16.1 Flexibility tests

- Tick the box corresponding to your movement range following the guidelines listed below.
- Perform a thorough warm-up before measuring your flexibility.
- Hold each stretched position for 3 seconds before measuring.
- Do not bounce into the movement.
- Average values will vary with body size and body type.

Test	Poor	Average	Good
Keep your straight leg on the floor and pull your bent knee towards your chest.	knee further than 15 cm from ribcage	knee 10–15 cm from ribcage	knee to ribcage
Keep the soles of your feet together and press your knees downwards towards the floor.	more than 15 cm from floor	15 cm from floor	less than 15 cm from floor
Keep the knees locked and reach forwards towards the toes.	more than 15 cm from toes	10–15 cm from toes	touching toes

231

Table 16.1 Flexibility tests cont.

Test		Poor	Average	Good
The lower leg is bent and held still, the top leg lowers towards the ground.		above horizontal	horizontal	below horizontal
	Stand 50 cm from a wall. Lean forwards, keeping the feet flat on the floor and the knees locked.	more than 60 degrees	60 degrees	less than 60 degrees
Keep the forehead and chest on the ground and lift the straight arms upwards.		less than 15 cm from floor	15–20 cm from floor	more than 20 cm from floor
	Reach behind the back and try to grip the fingers of the opposite hand.	fingers more than 15 cm apart	fingers 10–15 cm apart	fingers touching

Table 16.1 Flexibility tests cont.

Test	Poor	Average	Good
Keep the arms straight and try to cross them over as far as possible.	cross at wrist	cross at elbow	cross at upper arm
Keep the foot flat on a stool and press the knee towards the wall.	more than 50 degrees	40–50 degrees	less than 40 degrees
Keep the knees together and bent to 90 degrees. Allow the heels to drop outwards.	less than 70 degrees	70–90 degrees	more than 90 degrees
Lock the arms flat out and measure the distance between the pelvic crest and the floor	more than 15 cm from floor	15–10 cm from floor	less than 5 cm from floor

Table 16.1 Flexibility tests cont.

Test	Poor	Average	Good
Keep the arms flat on the floor and twist the trunk to allow the knees to lower towards the floor.	more than 10 cm from floor	10 cm from floor	touching floor
Keep the small of the back touching the chair back and flex the spine (not the hips) maximally.	fingers to mid-shin	fingers to floor	flat hand to floor
Keep the feet flat and the knees locked. Without leaning forwards or backwards reach down the side of the leg.	fingers above knee	fingers to knee	fingers below knee
Keep both legs straight and flex one hip as far as possible.	less than 90 degrees	90 degrees	more than 90 degrees

Table 16.1 Flexibility tests cont.

Test		Poor	Average	Good
	Abduct both legs while keeping the small of the back flat and the legs straight.	less than 90 degrees	90 degrees	more than 90 degrees
		heel further than 10 cm from buttock	heel 5–10 cm from buttock	heel to buttock
Keep the knees together and flex one knee maximally.				
	Keep the knees and ankles together throughout the test. Slowly sit back on to the heels. Measure the distance between the top (dorsum) of the foot and the ground.	greater than 5 cm	5 cm	flat

RELIABILITY

Reliability is really the consistency of the results obtained from a series of tests. We can talk about reliability in terms of observed score, true score and error score. When we measure range of motion with a goniometer, for example, we are not measuring the real joint angle, because the goniometer is attached to the skin and not to the bones. What we are seeing is an observed score. If we were to X-ray the moving joint and measure the bones directly, we would obtain the true score. The difference between these two, the real range of motion and the apparent range of motion, is the error score.

The error in a measurement may come from four main sources:

- Subject errors include things such as motivation, fatigue and health. If, in our study, an individual injures their hamstrings, this will affect their flexibility and, therefore, the test results. Equally, a subject who is less motivated may not pull the limb as far as they would if they were practising an active stretch.

- Test errors may occur through lack of practice and familiarity with the results, as well as through technique and lack of attention to detail. When a tester knows the value of a result, they may be able to influence it by over- or under-estimating a measurement. Equally, a poor standard of testing through lax positioning of a goniometer, for example, may produce considerable error.

- Scoring error is due to the selection of inappropriate measurement values, for example measuring joint movement in single inches rather than degrees.

- Instrumentation error results when instruments are not calibrated, or they simply break down – something that happens all too often.

RELIABILITY AND TESTERS

An additional aspect of reliability concerns the variation of the results obtained for a test from day to day, or between two people performing the same test. This is especially important if we are using a test to measure progress or to assess the effectiveness of a particular fitness or rehabilitation programme. For example, if tester A measures the flexibility of a subject's hamstrings using a straight leg raise (SLR) test today, will they use exactly the same test when they test again tomorrow, or next week? This is called intra-tester (or intra-rater) reliability, and is a measure of the consistency or repeatability of a particular measure. The more complex a test,

the less reliable it is likely to be, because it will be easier to make mistakes when applying the test. Alternatively, tester A uses the SLR test to measure a subject's hamstring flexibility, and for the next workout tester B uses the same test on the same subject, are both testers applying the test in exactly the same way? This is called inter-tester (inter-rater) reliability.

To improve both intra- and inter-tester reliability, the tests that we use should be agreed by everyone so that we all apply them in the same way. Also, if we are measuring parts of the body, it is better to base our measurements on bone rather than skin and muscle (soft tissue), as bone is less likely to change or vary. Soft tissue can swell, build up with strength training, waste with disuse etc., whereas bone will not. For this reason, we use the pieces of bone that are close to the skin's surface as the points to measure. These are called 'bony landmarks', and some are listed in table 16.2.

Table 16.2	
Landmark	**Position**
• Lateral malleolus of tibia	• Outside bone of ankle
• Head of the fibula	• Outside bone of knee splint bone
• Lateral epicondlyle of femur	• Outside upper knee
• Greater trochanter	• Outside upper thigh/hip
• Anterior superior iliac spine	• Point on outside/upper pelvis
• Posterior superior iliac spine	• Dimple at upper tailbone
• Acromion process	• Point at end of collarbone

MEASURING FLEXIBILITY IN THE LABORATORY SITUATION

A number of methods is used to measure changes in flexibility which occur in research studies, and the methods vary depending on the flexibility feature being studied. Where the straight leg raise (SLR) action is being studied, the range of motion and the resistance to motion may be studied using an isokinetic dynamometer.

This method of measuring SLR using a machine (instrumented) rather than the therapist's hands (manual) is called the instrumented straight leg raise or iSLR. Both range of motion (excursion angle) and muscle stiffness may be measured. The pivot point of the machine arm is aligned with the hip joint (normally taken as the centre of the greater trochanter) and the non-active leg, pelvis and trunk are secured with straps to prevent compensatory movement. The lumbar spine is supported using a pad to prevent the lumbar lordosis from flattening. As both the hamstrings and sciatic nerve are placed on stretch during this movement it is essential that the same ankle angle is used in all testing so that a greater or lesser stretch is not placed on the nerve in one movement but not in another. Generally the ankle is fixed at 90 degrees for consistency. For each subject the leg is moved passively by the dynamometer, which moves at a set rate and records the resistance offered by the stretching muscle at end range. Stretch tolerance is measured using a visual analogue scale (VAS).

Muscle stiffness may be recorded as maximal, that is the maximum torque (measured on the isokinetic dynamometer) which the subject can tolerate, and passive stiffness, which is the force required to lift the leg, again given as a computer reading by the machine.

Using an intensive four-week programme of passive stretching exercises consisting of three sets of 30-second hold for hamstrings and gluteals

Definition:

An *isokinetic dynamometer* is a computerised machine which provides reliable measurement of muscle force for assessment and can be used to produce controlled movements for rehabilitation. The machine can measure isometric (contract and hold), concentric (push), eccentric (controlled lowering) and isokinetic (constant velocity) actions. Resistance offered by the machine varies throughout the motion range and so points of weakness can be determined. Generally machines of this type measure torque expressed in newton meters (Nm) and angular velocity expressed in degrees per second ($°S-1$).

Definition:

Force is the effect which one object has on another, for example a push or pulling which causes the leg to move. *Torque* is a force which causes a turning action. In the case of the iSLR it is the force which causes the hip joint to rotate.

(15-minute duration per session, five days per week), Marshall et al., (2011) found that muscle extensibility measured as motion range increased by 20.9 per cent and passive stiffness reduced by 31 per cent. Interestingly, this result differed from others which had shown no change in passive stiffness through stretching, and the authors of this 2011 study argued that the intensity of the stretching programme was a deciding factor for producing the clinical effect.

Before stretching

After stretching

Figure 16.7 Ultrasound scan

The effects of stretching exercises on muscle local ultrastructure can be studied using a real time ultrasound scanner (ultrasonography).

The scan above (figure 16.7) shows a muscle seen via an ultrasound scan. The muscle fibres and tendon sheets (aponeurosis) can be seen as white linear areas on the black background.

Looking at stretching of the gastrocnemius muscle, Samukawa et al., (2011) studied displacement of the musculo-tendinous junction (MTJ) between the superficial and deep aponeurosis of the medial belly. Pennation angle (angle the muscle fibre makes with the deep aponeurosis) was also measured, as was fascicle length (*see* chapter 2 for details of aponeurosis). Where stretching changes the muscle architecture the fascicle length would increase and the pennation angle reduce, indicating that the muscle itself had lengthened. Where the MTJ moves, without changes to the muscle architecture, it is likely that lengthening has occurred within the tendon rather than the muscle. In the case of the Samukawa (2011) study, MTJ change was seen without alteration in muscle architecture as measured above.

SUMMARY

- We need to measure flexibility to know the current level of a client's movement range.
- Measuring flexibility enables us to judge if any muscle imbalance exists and then to chart a client's progress.
- Flexibility can be measured using score charts, measuring devices (goniometers) and photographs.
- Angles obtained during measurement are compared to normal values and to the other side of the client's body.
- Measurements may appear accurate when, in fact, they are not. Exercises that combine movements of two body parts simultaneously must be checked closely.
- Validity asks, 'Does a test measure what it claims to do?', while reliability asks, 'Was each test of a batch the same?'

STRETCHING AND SPORTS INJURIES

17

TISSUE HEALING

If you slip on a pavement and sprain your ankle, your body reacts immediately by starting a healing process. This process can be divided into three phases: inflammation, proliferation (sometimes called regeneration), and remodelling.

INFLAMMATION

Following injury, the inflammatory phase lasts between four and six days. The appearance of the body at this time reveals four classic signs: redness, swelling, heat and pain, which together lead to a loss of function in the injured body part (*see* fig 17.1).

- Redness: When tissues tear, small blood vessels are ruptured, releasing blood into the surrounding area. Injured tissue cells die and chemicals are released, irritating the local tissues and causing local blood flow to increase. This leads to the red appearance.
- Swelling: Changes in the concentration of fluids around the blood vessels cause watery fluid to leak out of them and into the surrounding tissues, giving rise to swelling. If the injury is close to the body surface, for example an injured ankle ligament, the swelling is readily apparent; if the injury is deeper in, however, the swelling may not be seen on the body surface, but only felt as pressure and stiffness.
- Heat: Increased metabolic activity from the inflammation causes heat, which is felt over the skin surface.
- Pain: The combination of pressure from the swelling and chemical irritation from metabolic products causes pain.

With a minor injury, the inflammatory phase may end in three days, but with more serious injuries, inflammation can remain active for five or six days. When an injury occurs and the tissues tear, their tensile strength (capacity to stretch) immediately drops (*see* fig 17.2). During the inflammatory phase, the strength of the injured

Figure 17.1 The signs of inflammation

239

tissues relies on clotted blood and tissue fluids, so the injured area is very weak. Until the blood and swelling clears and new collagen tissue forms (see below), the tensile strength of the area remains poor. During this time, we say that the tissues are in their 'lag' phase where, although healing is progressing, tissue strength remains unaltered. Any stretching applied at this stage can easily disrupt the healing process and prolong the inflammation, making the total healing time longer.

> **Key point:**
>
> The time from injury occurring to the beginning of the formation of strong collagen, which bridges the injured area, is about three to five days. Do not stretch before this time as the tissues are too weak.

> **Key point:**
>
> Gentle exercise strengthens the collagen tissue bridge, which forms as part of the healing process.

Figure 17.2 Tissue strength following injury

PROLIFERATION

Following inflammation, proliferation occurs. Within the injured area, the cells that were supplied by the damaged blood capillaries will have died, and these must be removed if healing is to be effective. Removal of dead cells is the job of special blood cells that engulf the dead material and digest it. Once this has occurred, new capillaries start to grow into the damaged area, forming delicate granulation tissue. By the third to fifth day after injury, a special form of tissue called collagen (*see* page 201) has started to form; this material will join the damaged tissues by forming a 'bridge'.

The collagen fibres are laid down haphazardly and, if this orientation remains, the scar formed will be very weak. To improve the strength of the scar, gentle movement should be performed, which will stretch the healing collagen fibres and cause them to line up in the direction of stress

applied, making the eventual scar far stronger. The size of the collagen fibres also depends on regular movement: with exercise, larger and stronger fibres form and the fibres bond to each other, further increasing the tissue strength. Exercise, correctly prescribed, will therefore create a stronger and more suitable healing breach across injured tissues (this is represented by the dotted line on the graph shown in figure 17.2). Most of the collagen will have been laid down by 16 to 21 days after injury, so this is the time when stiffness will be greatest and stretching will be most effective.

REMODELLING

About 21 days after the injury, the remodeling phase begins. During this phase, the amount of collagen produced is equal to the amount broken down. Although the total amount of collagen

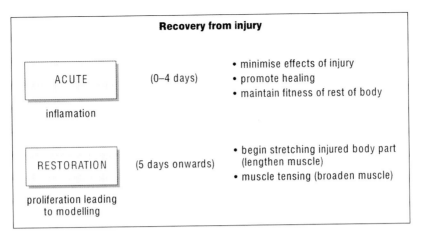

Figure 17.3 Acute and restoration phases of an injury

remains the same, the fibres overlap and form a mat of adhesions, which will stick to the surrounding tissues if movement is not performed. The collagen will also begin to shrink unless stretching exercises are continued. The function of this phase of healing is to make the healing bridge as similar as possible to the tissue that was injured. Although the tissue bridge will not look exactly like the injured tissue, its function will be similar. For this reason, exercise is vital. Without exercise, the bridge ends up tight and short, restricting normal movements and sometimes causing changes in alignment.

TIMESCALE FOR STRETCHING

As we discussed above, it is clear from the effect on healing that stretching is not appropriate immediately after injury for the following two reasons. First, the injured area is very weak and easily disrupted. Any amount of stretching could easily pull it and increase the tissue damage, which in turn will re-start the inflammation. Second, collagen tissue will not begin to form until the dead material produced by the injury is removed, so until that happens there is nothing there to stretch. We can divide the post-injury period into two distinct phases (*see* fig 17.3).

ACUTE PHASE

The first is the acute phase, from the day of injury to four days after. During this time the area is still inflamed, and our aim should be to minimise the effects of the injury. This can be achieved by using ice or cold water to slow down the metabolic rate (the amount of tissue activity), and reduce cell death from the low amount of oxygen present in the area. Swelling should be contained by using an elasticated bandage, and the fitness of the rest of the body should be maintained by using exercises that do not stress the injured area.

RESTORATION PHASE

After four or five days the inflammation will have subsided, and we enter the restoration phase. Stretching is needed to ensure that the collagen fibres of the injured tissue strengthen and face in the right direction to support the body part. Strengthening exercises must also be performed to tense and broaden the muscles. This moves the muscle fibres apart and prevents them from sticking together.

CLASSIFICATION OF INJURY

When muscles are injured, we say they are *strained*; when ligaments are injured, they are *sprained*. Both strains and sprains can be categorised into grades that represent the severity of the injury and the amount of tissue that has been damaged.

LIGAMENT INJURIES (SPRAINS)

Three grades of ligament injuries are used. Grade I sprains involve only slight tissue damage and the area is tender to touch, swelling is only slight and the body part moves almost normally. With grade II sprains, more ligament fibres are injured, local pain is more intense and movement is more limited. Grade I and II injuries are common when, for example, the ankle is twisted. Grade III injuries are far more serious because they involve complete rupture of the tendon. A skiing injury is a typical example of this type. There is considerable pain and swelling, and it is impossible to take the bodyweight through the injured limb. These injuries often require surgery to repair the ruptured ligament, followed by intensive physiotherapy.

MUSCLE INJURIES (STRAINS)

Muscle strains can be classified into four grades. Grade I (mild) strains involve tearing of only a few muscle fibres and subsequent local bruising.

The area feels stiff for a few days and then clears up fairly quickly. Grade II (moderate) strains are more severe. A larger number of muscle fibres are injured, and injury occurs over a greater area. The muscle membrane (fascia) still remains intact, so bleeding is contained within the muscle and forms what is called an *intramuscular haematoma*. The area again feels tight, but this time a local raised area is felt over the bruising and the muscle gives pain when tensed or stretched. A pulled hamstring is an example of a grade I or II muscle strain. With grade III (severe) strains, a larger area of muscle is affected. The muscle fascia is partially torn, and more than one muscle may be involved. Bleeding is more profuse, and it spreads over a larger area: because the muscle fascia has torn, blood spreads throughout the area, causing skin discoloration. A typical example here is a 'dead leg', where bruising spreads from the injured thigh down into the knee and calf. The grade IV injury is a complete rupture. The muscle-ends contract and a distinct gap can be felt between the injured muscle fibres. In some cases, a snapping sound may have been heard at the time of injury. Bleeding and swelling are considerable, and the muscle cannot be tensed up. This type of injury may require hospital treatment.

The classification of an injury is a guide to the period of rest and the amount of stretching that is required. As a general rule, the stretching should not be painful, but you should feel that it is lengthening the muscle. Never force a stretch, and never exercise through increasing pain. If something is painful, and the pain goes away with stretching, that is fine. However, if the pain starts to increase, the stretch should be stopped.

STRETCHING EXERCISES FOR INJURIES

The following stretches are for general guidance only. If you suffer a sports injury, see a physiotherapist. The sooner an injury is seen, the better; if left without treatment, injuries can put you out of sport for far longer. In addition, minor aches and pains are often signs that something is going wrong with the body. If this is caught in time, a more severe injury can often be prevented.

THE SPRAINED ANKLE

When you sprain your ankle, the most common injury is to a portion of the lateral ligament on the outside of the joint. This tissue limits plantarflexion, inversion and adduction of the foot. The easiest way to stretch this area is to cross the injured leg at the shin over the uninjured one; one hand steadies the lower leg on the injured side, while the other is cupped around the foot and ankle to pull it down, round and inwards. The stretch should be gentle and static.

Once this has been achieved, the next stage is to stretch the ankle actively by standing and rocking over on to the outer edge of the foot, or by walking on an inclined surface. This movement is controlled, but eventually faster actions must be used to develop agility in the ankle structures. This can be achieved by walking on an uneven surface such as soft ground or sand.

You can also make your own uneven surface by placing four or five cushions on the ground and walking, and then slowly jogging, over them in bare feet. At each stage, the action must be controlled so you don't feel that the movement is 'running away' with you.

As well as stretching the side of the ankle, walking on an uneven surface also strengthens the muscles surrounding the ankle so that they can support or 'stabilise' the joint. This function of ankle stability is the most important aspect of fitness to develop following an injury. Another way to work on stability of this type is to stand on one leg (the injured one) and hold this position for 20–30 seconds. When you do this, you will notice all of the muscles around the ankle 'flickering' as they work hard to stabilise the joint.

Key point:

Following a sprained ankle, stretch the outside of the joint using a plantarflexion and inversion movement and stabilise the joint using single leg standing.

SHIN SPLINTS

Shin splints is a condition affecting the shin muscles, which are contained within compartments running alongside the tibia and fibula. With training, the muscles swell and thicken and, as this happens, the pressure within them increases. Because the muscles are contained within an inflexible compartment, they cannot bulge outwards; therefore, they bulge inwards, cutting off their own blood supply. It is this reduction of blood flow and the build-up of acids within the muscles that causes pain. Stretching exercises can help some types of shin splints by preventing the muscles becoming short and tight.

On the front of the shin, the anterior compartment contains tibialis anterior and the toe extensors (*see* fig 17.4). These muscles pull the foot and toes up into dorsiflexion. To stretch them, we have to press the foot slowly

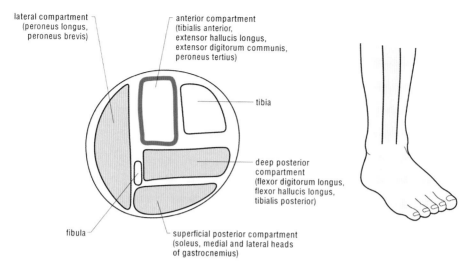

Figure 17.4 Compartments of the lower leg (Norris, 1998)

into plantarflexion immediately after running. We begin by kneeling with the feet flat on the ground. From this position we sit back on to the heels, pressing the feet into plantarflexion. To increase the stretch on the toes, place a folded towel on the floor beneath the toes to press them into flexion. Hold the position for 30–60 seconds to allow the muscles to 'give' gradually. Repeat the stretch 5 times after each run.

THE PULLED HAMSTRING

When you tear a hamstring, you may injure the muscle in its centre part (belly) or at the musculo-tendinous (MT) junction – the point at which the hamstring joins to the bones of the pelvis, or the knee, via the muscle tendon (*see* fig 17.5). The difference between these two areas is that the MT junction does not contract, while the muscle belly does. As well as stretching, muscle-belly tears will need strength training to broaden the muscle and separate the muscle fibres to prevent them sticking together. Injury to the MT junction often responds to stretching alone.

Because the hamstrings work over the hip and the knee, two types of stretches are necessary. First,

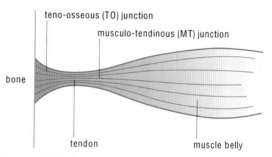

Figure 17.5 Areas of injury in a muscle

the muscle must be stretched with the leg straight (see exercise 3, page 105). Then, once adequate flexibility has been regained, the elastic strength of the muscle must be worked on. First stretch the muscle, then contract it rapidly from this lengthened position. To do this, lie face-down on a bench with the injured leg over the bench side so that the hip is flexed to 90 degrees. A small (3 kg) weight is attached around the ankle. From the stretched position, the hip is extended to pull the leg upwards against the resistance of the weight (*see* fig 17.6(a)). The movement can be modified to use both the knee and the hip by training with a partner. The partner provides the resistance by pushing on the heel, and

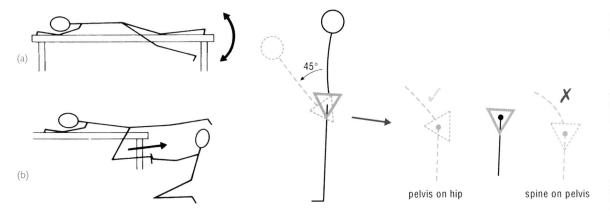

Figure 17.6 (left) Combining strength and stretch of the hamstrings: (a) hip extension over side of bench; (b) combined knee and hip extension against partner's resistance; (c) sprint jumping.

Figure 17.7 (above) Hip hinge action

the movement starts with the knee and hip both flexed to 90 degrees. From here, extend both the hip and knee simultaneously against resistance, hold the maximally contracted position for 1–2 seconds, and then lower the leg while maintaining tension in the muscle (*see* fig 17.6(b)). This controlled action progresses to spring jumping actions (*see* fig 16.6(c)), moving from a flexed hip/knee position to a fully extended position.

To work the upper part of the hamstrings and the gluteals, we have to perform a posterior pelvic tilt against resistance. Functionally, the action involves lifting, so this can become a useful exercise. The action is called a 'hip hinge' or 'good morning' exercise (*see* fig 17.7). Begin by standing with your legs straight and a stick across the shoulders. Keeping the legs and back straight, bend forwards from the hips to 45 degrees, and then return to standing. The action must move from the hip as a pivot rather than from the lumbar spine: moving from the lumbar spine will dangerously overstretch the lumbar tissues.

In sport, the hamstring muscles work with a 'whipping' action, often stretching rapidly. In order to be sport-specific, our stretching programme must reflect this, so dynamic stretching (*see* page 59) is required. For this, exercise 118 (Leg swing – forwards and backwards, *see* page 173) is used. Swing the leg progressively to shin, waist and then chest level, beginning slowly and gradually building up speed. Once you are confident with this single plane (flexion-extension) action, change to a multi-plane movement, kicking across the body (extension-abduction to flexion-adduction)

Key point:

The hamstrings perform fast whipping actions in sport and work over two joints. Begin with slow static stretching and build to dynamic stretching, using single- and two-joint activities.

and build in rotation movements. The final stage of progression is to use sports actions (such as kicking a football) as exercise. Begin with a slow gentle tap and build to a rapid kick, aiming to cover a large distance.

THE SWOLLEN KNEE

When the knee suffers a minor injury, it will swell and limit the movement of the joint. As the swelling clots and the injury heals, both the physiological movements and the accessory movements of the joint will be limited. This means that the joint will lose its normal movement and its healthy springy feeling (joint play). Stretching into flexion and extension will help you to regain the physiological movements, but the accessory movements will only return if these actions are combined with stresses to the knee that apply rotatory and shearing forces. These will work on all aspects of agility, and also help to build 'confidence' in the knee.

Start by standing with the feet shoulder width apart, then step forwards and across with the uninjured leg so that the stress is taken on the injured knee. Step backwards and across to place the opposite stress on the joint (*see* fig 17.8(a)). This action can be used as a side-step to perform a 'grapevine' action. Bending the knee further will increase the stress on the knee, and performing the action over a bench to bend the knee to near maximum will test the knee fully (*see* fig 17.8(b)). Because these actions stress the knee considerably, they must be carefully controlled.

When the rotation movement of the knee is limited, particularly after injury to the inner ligament (medial collateral ligament), this can be regained by twisting the tibia on the femur. A simple exercise is to place the foot up on a swivel chair so that the knee and hip are flexed to 90 degrees. Turn the chair by twisting the tibia and foot. As the foot moves outwards, the tibia

(a)

(b)

Figure 17.8 Developing agility in the knee: (a) 'grapevine' movement to place sideways strain on knee; (b) increasing range of movement

is externally rotated and the medial ligament is stretched. Gentle stretching of this type will make the ligament stronger by stressing and relaxing it to help the ligament fibres line up in the direction of the stress on the knee.

THE 'KICKING' MUSCLE

Injury to the rectus femoris or the 'kicking muscle' is common in football. The injury usually occurs either when an ineffective warm-up has been performed, or towards the end of the game when fatigue sets in. Either way, stretching is needed to restore the length and spring of the muscle. Passive stretching is performed by simultaneously flexing the knee and extending the hip. Once the same range can be achieved on both the injured and the uninjured side, the elastic strength of the muscle must be worked on. The action is to move from a fully stretched position to a fully contracted position of hip flexion and knee extension. This is performed against a resistance, which can be supplied by an elastic band, by a low pulley in a weight training room or by a training partner (*see* fig 17.9).

(a)

bench

resistance band

(b)

Figure 17.9 Stretch-contract of the rectus femoris: (a) fully stretched position (hip extension and knee flexion); (b) fully contracted position (hip flexion and knee extension)

Figure 17.10(a)
Hip adductor stretch for groin strain

Figure 17.10(b)
Hip adductor stretch for groin strain

GROIN STRAIN

Groin strain is also a common injury in football, as well as in other sports that involve rapid sideways stretches of 45 degrees or greater while lunging or side-stepping. The adductor muscles of the hip attach to the lower part of the pelvis. The adductor longus, adductor magnus and adductor brevis all attach to the femur and have no action over the knee; the gracilis, however, attaches to the upper part of the inner surface of the tibia, so it can also flex the knee during certain actions. This is important, because adductor stretches must be performed both with the knee flexed to take the gracilis off stretch and tax the other adductors, and with the knee extended to stretch the gracilis itself. Two exercises are useful.

In the first exercise (*see* fig 17.10(a)), begin by sitting on the floor with the soles of the feet together. Holding the feet with the hands, press down on to the knees or thighs to force them into abduction.

The second stretch emphasises the gracilis. For this, lie on the back with the legs straight. Flex the right leg to 90 degrees at the hips, keeping it straight. From this position the leg is abducted, aiming to rest it on the floor (*see* fig 17.10(b)). Repeat using the left leg. In both exercises, PNF (contract–relax) stretching may be performed by lifting the legs against resistance (manual in the first stretch, gravity in the second) and then lowering the legs again to increase the range of motion. It is important for total rehabilitation of the adductor muscles following groin strain that strength training and stretching go hand in hand.

As the rehabilitation period progresses, fast explosive actions (plyometrics) must be built in. This can be done usefully in a swimming pool with breaststroke type actions and using elastic tubing in the gym. In addition, jogging, cutting, side stepping and zigzag running drills constitute

247

dynamic stretching and also prepare the muscle with sport-specific actions.

CLICKING HIP AND CLICKING KNEE

Clicking hip and clicking knee are two conditions that can result from tightness in the ilio-tibial band (ITB), the strong band of fascia that runs along the outside of the leg (*see* fig 17.11). At its top, the ITB attaches to the hip muscles and then passes over a knobble of bone at the top of the thighbone (femur) called the greater trochanter. As the leg is moved forwards and backwards, the ITB passes in front of and behind the trochanter. If tight, the ITB will flick over the trochanter like a guitar string. This causes pain and swelling, and often a clicking sensation that can be felt and, in extreme cases, actually heard. A similar mechanism exists at the knee, where the ITB can flick over a point of bone on the lower end of the thighbone called the lateral epicondyle. The painful clicking sensation that occurs here is often called 'runners knee'.

To reduce the chance of these conditions occurring, or to lessen the pain if they already exist, ITB stretching is used. Exercise 33, page 121, is designed to stretch the ITB by holding the pelvis still and adducting the hip. The position is held for 30–40 seconds, and initially only 3 reps are used. The movement should be performed daily.

The upper portion of the ITB at the hip may be isolated using exercise 32, page 121. Again,

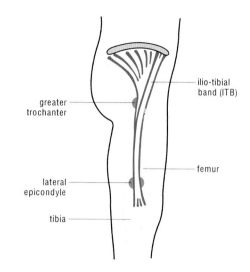

Figure 17.11 The ilio-tibial band (ITB)

the pelvis is held still while the hip is adducted. This time, however, the knee is bent, releasing the stretch in the lower portion of the ITB and throwing greater stress on the upper portion.

THE DEAD LEG

A 'dead leg' occurs when the quadriceps muscles of the thigh are severely bruised. This normally happens in rugby when a knee or head contacts the thigh at speed in a tackle. Blood vessels are ruptured and a large amount of blood is released into the muscle. The result is a large tense area within the muscle caused by a combination of blood and swelling. As the condition heals, the bruising tracks down through the muscle into the knee and calf. The athlete is unable to bend the knee because of tension in the quadriceps. The danger with this injury is that the release of blood can cause the area to calcify and form calcium bone salts within the muscle. If this happens it can be very serious, so stretching must be applied very cautiously under the supervision of a physiotherapist.

Initially, only active stretches should be used by lying on your front and simply flexing the knee through the power of the hamstrings alone. Once 90-degree knee flexion has been obtained, very gentle passive stretches can be performed by lying on your back and pulling the heel up towards the buttock. A towel placed around the ankle makes the reach easier. When the range of movement increases further and the pain and bruising subside, greater overpressure can be used to stretch the quadriceps by kneeling and sitting back on the ankles. These quadriceps stretches are described in exercises 18 (*see* page 114) and 25 (*see* page 177).

THE CALF AND ACHILLES

When the Achilles is injured, calf stretches should be performed with the knee flexed (see exercise 17, page 113); when the calf is injured, it is usually the long gastrocnemius muscle that is affected, and this should be stretched with the knee straight. When this can be performed statically without pain, the following active stretch is used.

Stand on a 5 cm block (or a thick book) and place the ball of the foot on the back edge. Allow the heel to lower down, keeping the knee locked: this will stretch the gastrocnemius. Starting from the standing position again, raise up on to the toes against your bodyweight. Initially, you should hold on to something to take some of your bodyweight off the calf. Eventually, full bodyweight can be used and the exercise can be speeded up until faster, more explosive actions are used to work the muscle for elastic strength.

THE ARCH OF THE FOOT

In sports such as the martial arts and some types of dance, which are carried out in bare feet or in very thin shoes, the amount of motion available to the big toe joint can overstretch one of the structures that forms the arch of the foot. This structure, the plantar fascia, can become inflamed or damaged. If this happens, stretching

should be employed once the injury has healed in order to restore flexibility. This can be achieved by plantarflexing the foot and flexing the toes simultaneously (see exercise 35, page 122). The plantar fascia will stand out as a tight cord in the sole of the foot.

STIFFNESS IN THE SPINE

There are many causes of back pain and for a full review of the subject the reader is directed towards Norris, Christopher M., *Complete Guide to Back Rehabilitation* (Bloomsbury, 2014). Here, we are concerned with stiffness in the back which may occur a day or two after training, or stiffness which has built up throughout the day and could limit sports performance. One of the main causes of back pain in general is repeated bending. This can occur in the low back through stooping, bending and lifting activities. In the thoracic spine it is the stooped sitting posture at an office desk which is the main enemy. We can use stretching exercises into extension to act as a mirror image of the flexion stress which has accumulated to give rise to the pain in the spine.

Repeated bending movements can squeeze the lumbar discs out of shape and increase the pressure within the disc (nucleus palposis). At either side of the spinal disc we have the facet joints which are synovial in nature (see chapter 2). These are the joints which click and pop when you move the spine rapidly and they will be placed under stress with rapid mis-timed movements in

> **Key point:**
>
> Repeated bending is a primary cause of back pain. Stretching into extension can be used to neutralise the effects of flexion stress accumulation.

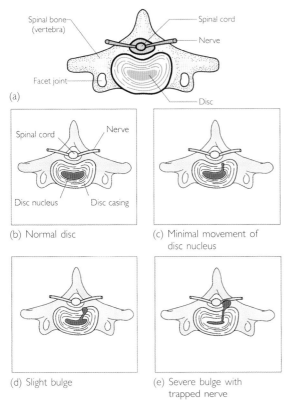

(a)

(b) Normal disc

(c) Minimal movement of disc nucleus

(d) Slight bulge

(e) Severe bulge with trapped nerve

Figure 17.12 The spinal disc and injury

sport. In addition, they can become swollen and inflamed in a similar way to any other joint in the body (*see* figure 17.12). Static stretching is useful to increase motion range by targeting the soft tissues but limiting the movement at the joints which may be inflamed. Dynamic stretches with their repeated nature place more stress on the joints within the spine but can have a positive pumping effect on the spinal discs.

Repeated bending movements cause the nucleus of the disc to become pressurised and press backwards towards the spinal nerves. Over time the nucleus can press through the outer casing of the disc and actually touch on to the nerve to trap it. When this happens pain radiates through

the buttock, down the leg, and into the foot. The nerve involved is the sciatic nerve and the condition is therefore termed sciatica. We can use *lower back extension – lying* (exercise 38, page 124) to regain some of the lost movement in the lumbar spine.

Stress on the facet joints often occurs in a lordotic posture (see chapter 5), but may also occur in sport through repeated extension movements or where extension is forced in a collapsing rugby scrum, for example. Now, the aim is to put flexion on the spine in a controlled manner and *lower back flexion – lying* (exercise 11, page 109) can help.

Stress on the thoracic spine through repeated sitting is one cause of the kyphotic posture covered in chapter 5. Here the stress is on the thoracic spine itself and the joints from the spine into the ribcage. In sport the same stresses can occur through posture which is exacerbated in racquet sports or throwing actions where thoracic flexion is increased or repeated. Thoracic extension movements such as *thoracic spine – over a roll* (exercise 128, page 179) or *thoracic spine – kneeling* (exercise 13, page 111) or *sitting* (exercise 14, page 111) can usefully target this condition.

Asymmetry of spinal rotation is common in racquet sports, which are obviously single handed in nature. Exercises such as *spinal rotation – using a stick* (exercise 130, page 180), or *spinal rotation – lying* (exercise 41, page 125) can be used to reduce stiffness but also to regain symmetry by performing more exercises on the stiffer side of the body.

THE RIBS

The ribs can be bruised or cracked, for example in a rugby tackle or when hit by the ball in hockey or cricket. When the injury has healed, stiffness often remains because the muscles between the ribs (intercostals) have tightened. To open the ribs and stretch the intercostals, we need to combine overhead reaching actions with deep breathing.

Twisting the trunk away from the painful area will increase the stretch still further. When performing this exercise, be careful not to take too many deep breaths without a rest, because this could cause you to hyperventilate and become light-headed. Perform the exercise three times and then breathe normally for 30–60 seconds before trying again.

THE FROZEN SHOULDER

When the shoulder is injured, it will swell and the joint capsule will fill with fluid. This will cause the capsule to tighten, eventually limiting the movement of the whole joint. Due to the shape of the capsule, certain movements will be limited more than others. In the case of the shoulder, lateral rotation (placing the hand behind the neck) becomes more limited and painful than medial rotation (putting the hand behind the back). The rotation movements can be regained by trying to touch the fingers together behind the back (exercise 135, page 181). Joint play can also be regained by holding on to an object and leaning back to pull the shoulder along its length and apply traction. Alternatively, sit sideways on a dining chair and hang your arm over the chair back. Place a thick towel over the chair back to pad the armpit area. Grasp something in the hand to provide a traction force, and pull down on the stiff arm with the other arm to give overpressure (*see* fig 17.13).

TENNIS ELBOW

In tennis elbow, the muscle most commonly affected is the one that extends the wrist (extensor carpi radialis longus). This muscle will become tight and must be stretched by flexing the wrist while keeping the elbow locked out. If the elbow is allowed to bend even slightly, the stretch will be taken off. A simple exercise is to stand facing a wall, and to straighten the elbow and keep it locked with pressure from the other hand. Place the back of the hand of the injured side against

Figure 17.13 Self-traction in the shoulder joint – hang arm over chair back

Figure 17.14 Stretching the extensor carpi radialis longus muscle in tennis elbow

the wall and lean forwards to press the wrist into flexion (*see* exercise 61, page 135). Performed correctly, this stretch can be felt up the whole arm and into the elbow.

Because the extensor carpi radialis longus also abducts the wrist, a further stretch can be placed on the muscle by adducting the wrist at the same time as flexing it. This is achieved by standing with the arm by the side, pronating the forearm and flexing the wrist (*see* fig 17.14). Take hold of the hand and press the wrist into further flexion and adduction, pulling the wrist towards the little finger (ulnar deviation).

Tennis elbow often involves the nervous tissues travelling through the elbow. The upper limb tension test movements described in chapter 16 (*see* page 233) are usually very relevant. Re-strengthening the forearm extensor muscles is also vital.

WRIST INJURY

Following a wrist injury, such as a severe sprain or fracture, most of the movements at the wrist will be limited. To regain these, three exercises are important. The first two are performed with the hand flat on a table top. Initially, the hand is placed palm down on the table surface, with the wrist crease at the table edge. The uninjured hand is placed on top of the injured one, and the elbow is moved up and down to produce flexion and extension of the wrist (*see* fig 17.15(a)). The leverage provided by the forearm, combined with the weight of the body provides overpressure at end-range for the static stretch.

For the second exercise, the hand is moved into the centre of the table so that the whole forearm is supported, and again the uninjured hand holds the injured one flat against the table surface. The elbow on the injured side is moved from side to side, sliding over the table surface to perform abduction and adduction of the injured wrist (*see* fig 17.15(b)). Finally, the arm is held at 90-degree flexion with the elbow close into the side of the body and the injured forearm supported by the cupped uninjured hand. A stick is held in the hand, and pronation and supination performed. Aim to move the stick into a horizontal position (*see* fig 17.15(c)).

FINGER INJURIES

Finger injuries are common in many sports and are caused either through trauma, for example in martial arts and football, or from overuse, for example in rock climbing. Where swelling is profuse, movement can often become limited very quickly, so stretching is vital. As the structures of the hand and fingers are very delicate, the stretching should be applied 'little and often' as a general rule. Three or four shorter bouts per day are better than a single long bout.

The movements are flexion, extension and abduction, all performed with manual overpressure. For flexion, the finger is bent to its maximal extent, and then gripped on the proximal and distal phalanx. Pressure is exerted to try to bring the fingertip to the underside of the knuckle. With extension, the movement must

Figure 17.15 Wrist mobility exercises

be isolated to each individual joint. One finger is placed proximal to the joint to fix it, while the other is placed distal to the joint to force the movement. For both of these movements, the exercise is best performed after soaking the hand and fingers in comfortably hot water for 15–20 minutes. Abduction is performed with the hand supported on a flat surface. The fingers are abducted and overpressure placed using two fingers of the opposite hand. The pressure is maintained for 20–30 seconds and then released.

SUMMARY

- Inflammation shows as redness, swelling, heat and pain.
- Proliferation is the stage of tissue regeneration.
- During proliferation, dead tissue is removed by white blood cells and new tissue forms. Controlled movement is needed to encourage correct tissue placement.
- When injured, ligaments sprain and muscles strain.
- Stretching forms a vital part of injury recovery.

SPORT-SPECIFIC STRETCHING

18

DESIGNING YOUR OWN PROGRAMME

In the majority of sports there is a central core of muscles that require stretching. Most sports involve some type of running action: this may be repeated running (marathon); single step running or lunging (badminton); or small bursts of speed (football). In each case the muscles used are similar, but the intensity of use and the range of motion will differ. While the running action forms the basis of motion, the throwing action frequently involves either a ball (throw and catch) or an implement used to strike an object (racquet or bat). Superimposed on these two basic sports movements are actions specific to the individual sports themselves. For example, the double-arm throwing action used in football differs considerably from the action of throwing the javelin, while the striking action of bat on ball in cricket is different from that of hitting a ball with a tennis racquet.

Therefore, to build up a comprehensive stretching programme for sports we need to choose exercises that cover both the core sports actions and the specific sports actions. By analysing which muscles are used in an action, we can estimate the patterns of muscle tightness that are likely to occur for each sport. Developing a stretching programme in this way can achieve two things. First, sports actions will be more efficient because we maintain a high range of motion. As we have seen on page 36, if a muscle is contracted from a comfortably stretched position, the amount of force achieved is greater than if a muscle is contracted from a shortened position. By stretching, we are therefore enhancing sports performance. Second, by preventing excessive shortening in general, and muscle imbalance in particular, we are maintaining optimal joint alignment. This provides a foundation for good biomechanics and balanced joint loading, increasing the likelihood of injury prevention.

MOVEMENT ANALYSIS OF CORE SPORTS ACTIONS

RUNNING

Running differs from walking in that when we walk we have at least one foot on the ground at all times; when we run we literally jump from

> **Key point:**
>
> Movement analysis provides us with an accurate baseline upon which to build a stretching programme.

foot to foot, so there is a stage when both feet are off the ground and the body is airborne. For this reason, running can be divided into two component phases, *stance* and *swing* (*see* fig 18.1). In the stance phase, the foot is on the ground and the body is decelerating. The muscles are working eccentrically to slow the body down and absorb shock through the whole of the lower limb. At the moment when the foot strikes the ground, the bodyweight is taken through the heel. As the bodyweight moves forwards, the foot flattens to absorb the shock, and finally the foot pushes with the toes to accelerate the body once more and propel it forwards. The forward action signals the start of the swing phase when the foot is off the ground. The limb is now accelerating and being catapulted through the air.

During heel strike, the anterior tibial muscles work to stop the foot slapping down on the ground, while the posterior tibials stop the foot from flattening too much. Tightness in either of these two muscle groups can be a cause of shin pain in runners. In mid-stance the knee is bent slightly and the quadriceps work to provide the spring in the legs, while the hip abductors support the pelvis and prevent it dipping down at the side. Tightness in these muscles at this stage of running is one cause of pain at the side of the leg and knee (or 'runner's knee'). As the heel rises and we begin to push off from the floor, the hamstrings rapidly extend the hip while the calf muscles plantarflex the foot. Both provide the thrust in running. If either muscle is tight, it is more likely to tear during sudden lunging or sprinting actions. During the swing phase, the hip flexors lift the leg through. These muscles may become tight and therefore more susceptible to injury, but usually any excessive tightness or shortness will affect the lumbar spine.

Stretches for running

Sports involving the running action will require calf, Achilles and anterior tibial stretches. In addition the hip flexors, hamstrings and quadriceps should be stretched, together with the abductors. Sprinting actions will require more attention to the hamstrings, while for kicking actions the rectus femoris will need stretching. Endurance running will need stretches for the ilio-tibial band (ITB) and anterior tibial muscles in particular, to protect against overuse friction injuries to these areas.

THROWING

In many sports the throwing mechanism is very similar. A baseball pitch and an overhead shot in tennis may seem very different, but both have three phases (*see* fig 18.2).

Initially there is the cocking phase, in which the arm is held up and back in preparation for the strike. The shoulder is abducted and externally rotated, the elbow flexed and the wrist

Figure 18.1 The running cycle (Norris, 1998)

(a)

(i) (ii) (iii) (iv) (v)

(b)

Figure 18.2 (a) The throwing action: (i) wind-up – athlete positions himself for the throw; (ii) cocking – lead leg moves forwards, arm moves backwards stretching body; (iii) acceleration – body drives forwards leaving arm behind; (iv) deceleration – object released, elbow continues to extend and shoulder to internally rotate; (v) follow through – trunk and lead leg show eccentric activity to dissipate energy; (b) similarity of throwing action to tennis serve (Norris, 1998)

extended. This position stretches the anterior shoulder structures and shoulder rotators and can place considerable stress on the medial ligament of the elbow. As the arm is pulled forwards into the striking position, it enters the acceleration phase. The body and shoulder lead the movement, coming forwards and leaving the arm behind, which pre-stretches the shoulder tissues. The shoulder flexors then contract rapidly with the shoulder rotators and elbow extensors to simultaneously bring the arm forwards and in. The acceleration phase takes place as a whipping action and so places considerable stress on the elbow structures. As the hand is flung forwards, the arm enters its final phase, the follow through. The object being thrown is released from the hand and the elbow extends rapidly. This places considerable stress on the bony knuckle of the ulna (olecranon process) as the elbow locks out.

Stretches for throwing

Sports involving any type of throwing action will require stretches to the anterior shoulder structures, the shoulder rotators and the elbow flexors. In addition, because of the single-arm nature of throwing, stretching must ensure symmetry between the two upper limbs.

MOVEMENT ANALYSIS OF SPECIFIC SPORTS ACTIONS

To know which additional stretching exercises are required, we need to analyse a particular movement used in a sport to find out which muscles it is affecting.

It is usually the muscles stretched by large movement ranges that we are concerned with, because these will be the ones needing stretching exercises: when throwing the javelin, for example, the shoulder and elbow of the throwing arm travel through extreme ranges so they will need stretching. The amount particular muscles are used must also be noted; those used powerfully are likely to shorten and require additional stretching. For example, the pectorals and anterior deltoids are used powerfully when performing bench press actions in weight training, so they tend to become very short.

Postures used in a sport are also a clue to the stretches that may be needed. Prolonged activity in a particular posture will cause the body to adapt by lengthening muscles on over-stretched joints, and shortening those other joints not moved through an adequate range. In cycling, for example, the stooped position of the thoracic spine can give rise to stiffness and pain in this area.

The movement analysis process may be divided into four stages:

- **Stage one**: Initially, we look at the movement and decide in which plane the movement mainly occurs (*see* fig 1.14, page 18). This will give us an idea of the types of movement used. Abduction and adduction occur in the frontal plane, flexion and extension in a sagittal plane, and rotation in a transverse plane.
- **Stage two**: Once we have an idea of the type of movement involved in an action, we must decide which joints are moving and which remain still. For example, in a trunk movement, is the hip moving as well? Does the pelvis move on the spine or on the hip, or both?
- **Stage three**: After the joints, we consider the muscles that would ordinarily work to bring about the actions we have seen, for example the muscles that flex the hip. We then need to determine if these muscles are actually working during the sporting action we are looking at, and to do this we must palpate (touch) the muscle.

- **Stage four**: Finally, the fact that a muscle is working during a movement does not necessarily mean that it warrants stretching. To determine this, we need to know the range of motion (*see* page 18). It is only when a muscle is taken through a greater range than normal (full outer- and full inner-range, rather than simply mid-range) that we need to stretch it.

We will look at three examples from common sports to illustrate the movement analysis method: a football kick, a forehand shot in tennis and a golf swing when teeing off.

THE FOOTBALL KICK

When a kicking action is performed, the movement analysis is as follows:

- The movement occurs in both a sagittal plane and a frontal plane because the kick moves forwards and across the body.
- This movement will be flexion and adduction of the hip, extension of the knee and plantarflexion of the ankle.
- Some transverse plane motion may also be seen as the trunk rotates on the standing leg.
- The muscles involved in this action would, therefore, be the hip flexors and adductors, knee extensors and ankle plantarflexors. In addition, the abductor muscles of the standing leg will stabilise the pelvis to stop it from dipping, and the trunk muscles will control the trunk rotation brought about by the momentum of the swinging leg.
- The range of motion of both the hip flexors and adductors is greater than normal, as is the range of the plantarflexors. The twisting of the spine would only be greater than normal in a less active individual who is beginning or returning to play.

Key point:

To analyse a movement, determine (a) the plane of movement; (b) the joints moved; (c) the muscles stretched; and (d) the range of motion.

The stretching exercises to choose, therefore, would be for the hip flexors, hip adductors (including gracilis) and calf muscles. Exercises 7 (page 107), 8 (page 108) and 24 (page 117) would be appropriate.

THE FOREHAND IN TENNIS

In an average tennis forehand shot, the movement analysis is as follows:

- The left leg steps across the right to bring the body to face right (right trunk rotation).
- The right hand is raised (abducted and extended) to shoulder level with the elbow and wrist partially extending.
- The foot action is one of dorsiflexion, stretching the calf.
- The combination of trunk rotation and shoulder abduction/extension is usually rapid, though not of extreme range.
- Stretching exercises for the chest and shoulder should, therefore, be combined with power training for this area. The calf/Achilles and wrist extensors are taxed considerably in all racquet sports through repetitive actions, so they too will require stretching.

Exercise 85 (page 151) is appropriate for the chest/shoulder, while exercises 8 (page 108) and 61 (page 135) are useful for the calf/Achilles and wrist extensors.

THE GOLF SWING

In a typical golf swing (teeing off), the movement analysis is as follows:

- The body is angled forwards on the hips (pelvis anteriorly tilted on the hip) and the knees and hips are slightly flexed.
- The trunk is twisted (rotation) to the right on the semi-flexed leg.
- The arms are brought across the body to the right, raising the elbows to shoulder level and taking the hands over the right shoulder. To do this, the right shoulder externally rotates and the left internally rotates; these movements are reversed during the follow through.
- The trunk movement and the momentum of the combined body and club are taken through the semi-flexed knee and considerable rotation occurs, slowly during the wind-up, and then much more rapidly during the swing and follow through.
- The areas of concern are the combined movements at the trunk (flexion and rotation), which occur at speed and through considerable range, and the rotation at the knee. Both sets of movement are considerably greater than the normal movement ranges encountered in everyday life.

Trunk rotation stretches, pelvic tilt rehearsal and hip rotation movements are all important, with exercises 130 (*see* page 180) and 93 (*see* page 156) being appropriate. In addition, postural re-education may be required if an individual angles the body forwards through trunk flexion alone, with little movement of the pelvis on the hip.

SPORT STRETCHING CHARTS

The charts on the next page list five stretching exercises which may be used as part of a sport training programme for each discipline. Although these are useful stretches for each sport it must be remembered that each individual may have additional requirements determined by their body type, history of injury, and type or position of play. For each exercise refer to the exercise instructions before applying the stretch. Because these are basic foundation stretches, most have been chosen from chapters 7–9, and do not include partner, dynamic, neural or fascial stretches. Having practised the five stretches for 8–10 weeks and become proficient at them, you are encouraged to work with a coach or personal trainer to add more specialised stretching from chapters 10–14. You may also find it useful to swap one of your stretching periods for a yoga class to try a mind-body approach to your stretching.

Sport	Exercise				
Road running	4	9	18	22	17
Sprinting	5	7	12	19	23
Football	8	23	5	43	30
Squash	28	31	39	19	40
Tennis	5	20	47	57	68
Hockey	7	25	39	74	89
Golf	4	12	42	91	95
Cricket	43	9	14	74	10
Judo	43	48	59	74	79
Karate	6	57	74	79	93
Rugby	5	10	40	20	91

SUMMARY
- Running and throwing are core skills in many sporting activities.
- There are four stages to movement analysis: establishing the plane of movement, finding which joints have moved, determining which muscles are working and finding the range of motion.
- Perform the foundation stretching programme for your sport before adding more advanced stretches, taking into account your body requirements and sport position.

YOGA AS STRETCHING

19

WHAT IS YOGA?

The term yoga means union (yoke) and refers to the union between body, mind, emotion and breath. It is a system of exercise originally based on Hindu teaching, but nowadays a modified form of yoga is normally practised, which falls into the category of mind-body exercise alongside activities such as Pilates and t'ai chi for example. Yoga can be seen as mindful activity in that it combines both physical exercise and a mindfulness approach to movement. Participants are encouraged to pay attention to the feeling of their body during exercise with special attention to the breath. This concept of awareness of the breath is central to the mindfulness approach used in stress management (Williams and Penman, 2011). Classical yoga postures (asana) are linked to breath awareness and control (pranayama), concentration (dharana) and relaxation/meditation (dhyana).

A typical yoga class begins with a centring activity designed to act as a brake between the activities of daily living and the focus required in the yoga class. This would typically be a seated posture requiring the participant to close their eyes and focus on their breathing for example, thus turning their attention inward towards their body and away from environmental stimuli. The body of the yoga class uses exercises practised on a non-slip (sticky) mat and often uses basic

Definition:

Mindfulness is a psychological term inherited from the Buddhist tradition. It is paying attention to the present moment in a non-judgemental way.

props such as foam blocks, wooden bricks and webbing belts. Yoga exercises use a number of starting positions including lying, floor sitting, chair sitting, kneeling and both free- and wall-support standing. Exercises are usually practised individually but partner work can also be used.

Typically a yoga class will involve several postures progressing in intensity, and finishing with a relaxation and/or meditation session. The postures are often held for a number of seconds and clients are encouraged to relax and breathe normally during the postures. Postures are normally practised symmetrically with emphasis on good alignment as well as range of motion. In addition, counter poses are often used to prevent stress accumulation within the tissues. For example postures emphasising spinal flexion are often countered by those emphasising extension.

Body alignment when performing posture is usually compared to an idealised version typically presented by a yoga book, organisation or senior practitioner. Sometimes the reasoning behind the idealised postures lacks clear scientific evidence. Classical yoga usually claims that poses are passed down over the centuries from teacher (master) to pupil, and many organisations claim to represent the true postures. Scientific scrutiny has challenged the claim that all yoga postures are ancient and that the techniques are unchanged over millennia (Singleton, 2010). Where yoga poses are used as stretching exercises it is essential that an emphasis is placed on good body alignment using knowledge of anatomy, physiology and body mechanics.

YOGA POSTURES

Yoga postures (asanas) have individual names, which may describe the general body shape, an animal which the posture is said to resemble, or an individual after whom the pose is named. Poses have both Western and Sanskrit names, so for example Mountain pose is also called *Tadasana*, from the Sanskrit *Tada* meaning mountain and *asana* meaning posture.

ASANA PERFORMANCE

Several factors should be considered when performing a yoga asana (*see* table 19.1). Some of these concern body mechanics and are fairly universal to good exercise practice which underlies stretching. Others differ from standard exercise practice due to the mind-body nature of yoga. One of the similarities with modern practice is the use in yoga of *Bandhas* or body locks. These will be familiar to any exercise professional, although perhaps not in name. *Mula Bandha* (root lock) is essentially engaging the pelvic floor, *Uddiyana Bandha* (abdominal lock) the lower abdominal muscles, and *Jalandhara Bandha* (throat lock) the deep neck flexors through the use of a chin tuck action. Bandhas are often used during exercise

Definition:

Sanskrit is one of the original languages of the Indian sub-continent. Classical Sanskrit is rarely used nowadays except in traditional ceremonies in mainly Hindu and Buddhist practice. Versions of the language can be traced back to 1500 BCE.

to aid the firmness of a posture and to provide its root; expressions familiar to any exercise professional using core stability.

Good alignment is essential to yoga practice, and often props are used to allow an individual to perform a yoga pose even where they have physical characteristics which would limit them. So, for example, when reaching into a forward bend (Uttanasana) an individual with tight hamstring muscles is unable to touch the floor to take their bodyweight. Wooden yoga bricks may be used to bring the floor up to the student so they can take their weight on to their hands even though their flexion range is limited. Similarly in sitting forward bend (Paschimottanasana) an individual who cannot reach their feet can be given a yoga belt, and someone who cannot rest their head on to their legs a folded blanket to allow them to rest in a higher (less flexed) body position.

Yoga is described as a mind-body activity, and mindfulness is an awareness of body sensations and the breath as you practice the asanas. In traditional gym training there are often distractions which take a user's attention outside their body. Music, TV screens playing music videos and mirrors are all features which take the attention away from the body. By focusing on bodily sensations such as the firmness of a muscle or the precise position of the limb, as well as noticing the breath and the effect that this has on the posture, the attention is drawn within the user. Further, anxiety can occur in general life by constantly thinking of what the future may bring or regretting what the past has already brought. One of the aims of mindfulness meditation is to focus attention on the present moment. Again yoga can help with this by stressing to the user that they focus on the exercise stage they are in at the moment rather than being goal focused on the end result of an asana.

Focusing the attention on body sensation also aids proprioception. This can be further enhanced by the yoga emphasis on movement precision during practice. It is interesting to note that exercises which contain 'an intuitive search for elegance, pleasure and beauty' (Schleip and Muller, 2013) such as yoga, martial arts and dance have been found to be among the most effective at enhancing proprioception.

Yoga is obviously an exercise associated with stretching and a high degree of flexibility in practitioners. In addition to range of motion, the emphasis on extension of an asana is important. Reaching upwards and outwards to lengthen the body and limbs during a pose, and allowing unrestricted chest movement to facilitate unhindered breathing should be emphasised throughout yoga practice.

Table 19.1	Important factors in yoga practice
Factor	**Meaning**
Alignment	• Position of body parts relative to each other, and of the body relative to the floor or supporting surface. • Use supports such as yoga blocks/bricks/wedges/blanket/belt to improve alignment of pose. • Consider alignment at each stage of pose: going into, holding, and coming out of pose.
Extension	• Gradual lengthening (stretching) of body soft tissues. • Expansion and lift of chest. • Elongation of limbs to create space for movement to occur. • Extension occurs from the ground up.
Direction	• Connected to both alignment and extension, direction begins at the floor and moves through the body and limb.
Stability	• Holding the pose quietly (mindfully) with minimal muscle work, sensitivity and normal breathing. • Stability of the body centre (pelvic and/or shoulder girdle) for the limbs to move upon.
Precision	• Subtle adjustments to alignment to refine the pose. • An understanding of mental and emotional effects on asana practice (mind/body nature of yoga).
Mindfulness	• Focus attention internally to 'listen to the body'. • Aim to think in the present rather than focusing attention on the final exercise position (future) or being distracted by thoughts of daily activity (past).

(IYUK 2013, Kabat-Zinn, 2007)

Exercise 176 Mountain pose
(Tadasana)

Tips

Some individuals hyperextended their knees when they tighten the quadriceps muscles. To avoid this action, focus on maintaining a straight vertical line from your hips through your knees to your ankles. In addition, avoid over-arching your lumbar spine (hollow back posture) by gently drawing your abdominal muscles inwards and tailbone downwards.

For those with very tight, rounded shoulders it is helpful to practice the pose with your back against a wall. Focus on drawing the shoulders back to press against the wall (retraction) before reaching the fingertips downwards to the outer ankles.

Purpose

To teach standing body alignment is a preparation for further poses, and to increase appreciation of optimal posture.

Preparation

Begin standing with your feet together and hands by your sides, palms facing inwards.

Action

• Take your weight equally between your right and left foot, and between the toe and heel on each foot. Tighten your thigh muscles (quadriceps) to draw your knees straight and together. Lengthen your spine, reaching the crown of your head upwards, and draw your shoulder blades together slightly to open your chest. Straighten your arms, reaching your fingertips downwards towards your outer ankle bones (lateral malleolus). Maintain the position, breathing normally.

Exercise 177 Triangle (Trikonasana)

Purpose

To lengthen the side trunk and outer hip.

Preparation

Begin standing on a yoga mat with your feet approximately one leg length apart, toes facing forwards. Stretch your arms out sideways (shoulder abduction) keeping your elbows straight and palms facing the floor.

Action

- Turn your left leg outwards (lateral rotation of the hip) so that your toes face the short edge of the mat. Reach your left hand out and downwards placing it on to your left shin, while at the same time reaching your right hand upwards towards the ceiling. Avoid allowing the right side of your pelvis to roll forwards. Keep the pelvis aligned so that the hip joints are stacked (right and left joints aligned in a vertical position). Open your chest and extend your thoracic spine into a light shoulder retracted position. Reach with your right arm upwards and press with your left

hand on to your shin to come out of the pose. Repeat the action on the right side of the body.

- Perform a limited range action, taking the left hand down to a chair, placing your hand in the centre of the chair and keeping your arms straight. To increase range further, use a wooden yoga block placed with its long edge aligned vertically. The block should be aligned with your centre shin.
- To improve alignment, perform the pose with your back towards the wall, trying to press the upper pelvis backwards against the wall to maintain the stacked hip position.
- To reduce balance demand, perform the standard pose but keep your right hand on your hip, or place your hand behind your tailbone (sacrum) to encourage chest opening.
- To perform the revolved triangle pose (Parivrtta Trikonasana), begin with your feet wide apart and your arms stretched out horizontally in line with the long edge of a yoga mat. Turn your back (left) foot in well (60 degrees) and your right foot out fully (90 degrees) and at the same time turn your body to the right to bring your chest and outstretched arms to face the short end of your mat. Place your right hand on your hip and reach your left hand down to the floor on the outside of your leading foot. To maintain the alignment of your spine you may choose to place your hand on to a yoga block, your fingertips, or the flat of your hand depending on your flexibility. Finally, reach your right arm upwards, keeping it straight and pointing your fingertips to the ceiling.

Tips

The pose requires leg firmness and stability, with flexibility of the lateral trunk. The pose can be split into two portions, practising leg stability with the hands on the hips initially. Once acheived, the trunk movement and arm stretch may be practised.

Exercise 178 Warrior (Virabhadrasana)

Purpose

To build leg flexibility and strength in the legs while maintaining upper body alignment.

Preparation

Begin standing on a yoga mat with your feet wide apart (distance approximately 1½ leg lengths). Reach your hands out sideways so that your arms are straight, elbows locked and palms facing the floor.

Action

- Bend your left knee, pressing the knee forwards over the left foot and ensuring that the knee does not drop inwards into a knock knee position. Stop when the knee is at 90 degrees and your shin is vertical, thigh horizontal. Press on the left foot, straighten the leg and draw yourself back to standing, reverse the movement bending the right leg. This pose is *Warrior (II)*.

- Lower your arms and place your hands on to your hips. Turn your left leg outwards (outward rotation of the hip) to face your toes towards the short edge of the mat. Turn your trunk to the left, aiming to get your pelvis and shoulders facing the short edge of the mat. Bend your left knee, pressing the knee over the left foot. Stop when the knee is at 90 degrees and your shin is vertical, thigh horizontal. Reach both arms overhead keeping them shoulder width apart with your fingers straight, palms facing each other. Press on the left foot, straighten the leg and draw yourself back to standing. Reverse the movement bending the right leg. This pose is *Warrior (I)*.
- Perform Warrior (I), and from the final pose lower your trunk towards your left thigh and step in with your right foot. Press hard with your left leg and lift your right leg into a horizontal position keeping your thigh muscles tight. Reach forwards with your hands and aim to form a straight horizontal line from your hands through your shoulders, trunk and left leg. Release the pose by reversing the action. This pose is *Warrior (III)*.
- Both Warrior (I) and Warrior (II) may be performed as limited range motion poses, bending the knee only as far as is comfortable. To provide additional support the right hand may be placed on a chair when moving to the right. As leg strength increases, the knee may bend further until the 90-degree angle of the classical pose is obtained. Warrior (III) may be performed with the hands placed on a wall to aid balance and alignment.

Tips

There are three common errors which occur in the Warrior poses. The first is allowing the knee to drift inwards into a knock knee position. This places extra stress on the inside (medial aspect) of the knee. To prevent this, ensure that the knee passes over the centre of the foot. The second error is allowing the upper body to drop into a round shouldered position which restricts the chest and breathing. Avoid this by lengthening the spine, reaching the crown of the head upwards and keeping the chest open and the shoulders drawn back slightly. Finally, the training leg is placed on stretch (hip adductors), but must be active. If the leg is placed on stretch without quadriceps activity, the downward direction of the bodyweight can force the inside of the knee to overstretch (valgus stress) potentially damaging the inner (medial) knee ligaments. It is important therefore that the action of the trailing leg is to press against the yoga mat to lock the knee and lift the body upwards rather than allowing it to sag.

Exercise 179 Wide legged forward bend (Prasarita Padottanasana)

makes an angle of 90 degrees to your legs, place your hands on the mat directly beneath your shoulders.

- To increase the intensity of the stretch, bend your elbows and take your hands backwards to place them on the mat level with your feet. Keep your spine as straight as possible, aiming to place the crown of your head on to the floor.
- To reduce the intensity of the pose place your forearms on the seat of the chair placed in front of you, or place your hands on to wooden yoga blocks placed shoulder width apart on the mat in front of you.

Tips

As you angle your trunk forwards there is a tendency to flex the spine excessively. To avoid this, keep your hands on your hips and draw your elbows together to open your chest (retract your shoulder blades and extend your thoracic spine). To further reduce this tendency as you take your arms downwards, reach forwards and look forwards to maintain the extension of your thoracic spine.

Purpose

To lengthen the hip tissues (adductors and hamstrings) while maintaining lumbo-pelvic and upper body alignment.

Preparation

Begin standing on a yoga mat with your legs apart, feet facing directly forwards.

Action

- Place your hands on your hips and fold your body forwards keeping your spine straight and moving from your hip joints. When your trunk

Although this pose is practised on a sticky yoga mat, there is still a tendency for the feet to slip apart slightly. If you feel your feet slipping, you will naturally activate your hip adductor muscles to prevent this, increasing muscle tone and reducing the muscle's ability to lengthen into the stretch. To prevent foot slippage, work with a partner and place one foot against a wall, while your partner blocks your other foot with their own. Alternatively, link two yoga straps together and place these over your feet. Tighten the straps when your hips are in the abducted position to prevent your feet slipping outwards.

Exercise 180 Staff pose (Dandasana)

Tips

It is often useful in this pose to work with a training partner. Your partner can place the outside of their leg along the length of your spine, and gently draw your shoulders backwards, pressing your spine into a straight position against their leg. The action is to encourage rather than force the movement, and you must give feedback about what you are feeling in your back throughout the movement.

Purpose

To lengthen the hamstring muscles and rehearse a correct straight leg sitting (long sitting) pose.

Preparation

Begin sitting with your legs straight and spine upright. Your lumbar spine should be in its neutral position, but with a gentle inward curve (lordosis).

Action

- Place your hands on to the mat on either side of your hips and press down gently to extend your thoracic spine and lift your ribcage (sternal lift action).
- If you find it difficult to sit with your spine upright, sit with your back against a wall.
- If your spine rounds in the sitting position, sit on one or two foam or yoga blocks to anteriorly tilt your pelvis and realign your spine.

Exercise 181 Forward bend (Uttanasana)

Purpose

To lengthen the hamstring muscles, hips and spine from a standing position.

Preparation

Begin standing in mountain pose (*see* page 262).

Action

- Reach your arms forwards and then overhead, keeping your hands shoulder width apart. Angle your trunk forwards keeping your spine long and arms reaching in front of you to encourage thoracic spine extension. Reach forwards and downwards, moving your hands towards the floor. Place your hands on the floor and pause in this position, keeping your arms straight and thorax extended.

- For the final pose, reach your hands behind your heels and draw your trunk downwards on to your thighs. To come out of the pose release your hands from your heels and reach your arms forwards and upwards to extend your spine as you stand back to the upright position. Pause in mountain pose to recover.

- To reduce the intensity of the stretch reach your hands downwards on to wooden yoga blocks either placed on their long side (lower lift) or short side (higher lift). Where your hips are very stiff, begin the position with your feet shoulder width apart, and where your hamstrings are very tight, allow your knees to bend slightly (unlock or soften the knee) to partially release the pull of the hamstrings on to the pelvis and allow better lumbo-pelvic alignment.

- Where standing balance is impaired, the pose may be performed leaning against a wall. Stand back towards a wall with your feet slightly forwards. Position your sitting bones (ischial tuberosities) against the wall by anteriorly tilting your pelvis. As you move into the stretch, move your sitting bones up the wall.

Tips

This is an intense stretch of the hamstring muscles, and a high degree of hamstring flexibility is required to allow the pelvis to anteriorly tilt sufficiently to maintain spinal alignment. Where the hamstrings are very tight, anterior pelvic tilt is limited and movement downwards can only be obtained by increasing spinal flexion. Where excessive spinal flexion occurs it is important to reduce the movement range and maintain good overall body alignment rather than sacrificing alignment simply to reach further towards the ankles.

Exercise 182 Seated forward bend (Paschimottanasana)

Purpose
To lengthen the hamstring muscles, hips and spine from a sitting position.

Preparation
Begin sitting in the staff pose (*see* page 267), pressing your hands on to the floor to encourage thoracic extension and lifting of the ribcage.

Action
- Reach your hands forwards and then overhead keeping your arms shoulder width apart, to extend your thoracic spine. Maintain this thoracic extension and then reach forwards towards your feet, aiming to grasp your feet (knuckles outwards) and draw your upper body down on to your thighs.
- Where you are unable to reach your feet, loop a yoga belt around your feet (place the belt in the middle of the sole to avoid it slipping). Grasp the yoga belt with each hand and draw yourself forwards, aiming your lower ribs towards your thighs rather than your head to your knees. To encourage lift in your ribcage, move your elbows out to the side as you pull on the belt.
- This action may also be performed sitting on a chair where the pose becomes the same as the standing forward bend (Uttanasana) described on page 268.

Tips
If your hamstring muscles are very tight, or you have a tendency to hyperextended your knee, place a folded towel or yoga blanket beneath your knees. This will have the effect of bending the knee slightly (unlocking) to release the stretch in the hamstrings and tension in the posterior knee joint structures.

The exercise mimics the action of the sit-and-reach test (chapter 16) and your test score will improve with practice.

Exercise 183 Wide leg sitting (Upavistha Konasana)

Purpose

To lengthen the hamstrings and hip abductor muscles while maintaining an upright sitting posture.

Preparation

Begin in staff pose (*see* page 267), sitting on one or two yoga blocks to optimally align your pelvis and lumbar spine if required.

Action

- Lift each leg in turn to the side (hip abduction) ensuring that they are equidistant from the body mid-line. Keep the toes pointing upwards, avoiding outward or inward rotation of the hip, and maintain tension in the quadriceps muscles. Press your hands on to the floor and the side of your body to open your chest and lengthen your spine.
- Where you find it difficult to maintain spinal extension, use two yoga belts and loop them around the centre of each foot. Hold one belt in each hand and gently pull on the belts, retracting your shoulders and lifting your sternum.
- To provide further spinal support, perform the exercise with your back pressed against a wall.

Tips

To ensure that your pelvis is correctly aligned, you should be sitting on your sitting bones (ischial tuberosities) and pubic bone. Where you have begun the pose with your pelvis posteriorly tilted, place one hand under each ischial tuberosity in turn and pull backwards, drawing the buttock flesh (gluteal musculature) backwards.

Where you find you are unable to maintain spinal alignment, choose the *Hip adductors – wall support* exercise (page 117) instead. The actions are similar, but the whole body has been rotated through 90 degrees when using wall support rather than free sitting.

Exercise 184 Seated twist (Bharadvajasana)

Purpose
To release spinal stiffness by stretching the oblique abdominals and inert spinal tissues.

Preparation
Begin sitting side-on to a firm chair (yoga chair). Place your feet hip width apart and flat on the floor. Sit upright with your spine correctly aligned.

Action
- Turn towards the chair back and grip the top of the frame in each hand. Lift your elbows away from the sides of your body and place gentle overpressure on the chair to increase spinal rotation. Ensure that your shoulders remain horizontal throughout the action and you do not sideflex. Repeat the action facing in the opposite direction.
- You can also perform the pose kneeling, with a folded towel or blanket between your buttocks and heels to reduce the range of motion required at the knees. Turn to the right, placing your left hand on to the side of your right knee. Use your hands to encourage rotation range of motion and spinal lengthening.

- Perform the classical pose sitting on a foam yoga block. Bend your left leg placing your left foot to the outside of your left hip (hero or Virasana pose leg position). Bend your right leg placing your right foot inside your right thigh so that it passes beneath your left shin (cobbler or Baddha Konasana pose position). Readjust the position of the yoga blocks so that your hips are aligned horizontally. Turn your trunk to the right, pressing your left hand against your right knee and placing your right hand on the floor behind you.

Tips
The aim of this exercise is to use overpressure from the arms to encourage a greater range of spinal rotation. It is common to be asymmetrical with rotation being freer to one side than the other. With practice the motion range should become equal on both sides (symmetrical) and increase.

To use leverage to increase your movement range, perform *spinal rotation – using a stick* (*see* page 180).

Exercise 185 Lying straight leg stretch (Supta Padangusthasana)

Purpose

To lengthen the hamstring muscles, sciatic nerve and posterior fascia of the leg.

Preparation

Begin lying on a yoga mat on your back. Draw your right knee towards your chest and loop a yoga belt around the sole of your right foot, holding each end of the belt in either hand.

Action

• Keep your left leg straight and pressed against the floor by tightening your quadriceps muscles. Straighten your right leg by pressing your heel towards the ceiling, keeping your knee over your hip. Hold your leg in the vertical position for 10 – 20 seconds breathing normally. Hold the belt, pressing your foot against it, and retract your shoulders to avoid flexing your thoracic spine.

• Perform action one and gradually draw your straight leg into further hip flexion by reaching one arm straight overhead. At end range hold the position for 10 – 20 seconds breathing normally. Repeat the action with the left leg.

• Perform action one and transfer the belt to your right hand alone. Draw your leg out sideways into abduction keeping the foot in line with the hip. You may use your elbow against the floor as a point of contact. Aim to take the side of your foot towards the floor to avoid external rotation of the hip.

• Draw both knees towards your chest and loop a yoga belt around the soles of both feet. Straighten both legs, pressing your heels towards the ceiling to create a 90-degree angle at your hips (classical Urdhva Prasarita Padasana pose).

Tips

Each of these exercise sequences targets the posterior structures, with a different emphasis depending on the movement range and motion direction. Vary your practice to ensure all structures are covered.

Exercise 186 Downward dog (Adho Mukha Svanasana)

Purpose

To mobilise the chest, shoulders and hips while stretching the calf muscles and Achilles.

Preparation

Begin lying on your front on a yoga mat. Position your hands at the sides of your chest palms flat, and tuck your toes under, tightening your quadriceps muscles to straighten your legs.

Action

- Simultaneously press with your hands and feet, driving your hips upwards. Keep pushing until your arms are straight and level with your ears, and your hips are as high as possible. Tighten your quadriceps and calf muscles, lifting high on to your toes. Maintain this high pelvic position and gradually allow your heels to lower downwards, placing a stretch on your calves and Achilles.

Tips

Where you find it difficult to press with your arms, place your hands on to yoga bricks positioned against the wall to avoid slippage. The heel of your hands should be at the front edge of the block to provide purchase. The higher block position encourages greater activity from your arms. Where you are unable to lower your heels to the ground, place a block or folded blanket beneath your heels.

This exercise can also be performed as a partner action. For this your partner stands behind you, grips in front of your hips and draws your pelvis towards themselves, increasing the bodyweight you put over your heels. Where gripping the hip region is painful (or ticklish) use a yoga belt placed around your hips (at the level of the iliac crest) instead.

Exercise 187 Cobra (Bhujangasana)

spine throughout its full length. Initially, look in front of yourself and then towards the ceiling (cervical extension). Hold the upper position for three breaths and then lower to the mat under control.

Tips

The aim of this action is to move equally through the full length of the spine. As the thoracic spine is stiffer to extension than the lumbar spine, there is a tendency to focus the entire movement in the lumbar area. To discourage this, have your client visualise lengthening their tailbone and slightly posteriorly tilt their pelvis. However, ensure that the lower back and buttocks remain relaxed to reduce muscle tension in this area.

Purpose

To increase spinal extension range of motion.

Preparation

Begin lying on your front on a yoga mat with your feet together. Place your hands at the side of your chest with your palms downwards.

Action

• Begin the exercise by retracting and depressing your shoulder blades, and extending your thoracic spine to gradually lift your breastbone (sternum) from the mat. Press with your arms to continue the movement, extending your

Exercise 188 Plough (Halasana)

Purpose
To lengthen the posteriorly placed tissues and sciatic nerve.

Preparation
Begin lying on your back with your hands by your sides, palms downwards.

Action
- Draw your knees to your chest and press your hands on to the mat. Continue the movement, rolling your spine into flexion. Allow your legs to straighten, locking your knees and placing your toes on the floor. Bend your elbows to

support your spine with your hands on your upper back. As you release the pose, draw your knees back into your chest and place your straight arms on the ground. Lower your spine back on to the mat under control.
- To reduce the range of motion, place your toes on the seat of the chair rather than the floor. For additional support, place your shins on the chair seat padded with a folded blanket.
- Reduce the range of motion by performing the pose close to a wall, and rest your feet flat on the wall for support.
- Increase the workload on your shoulders by straightening your arms, interlacing your fingers, and pressing your straight arms downwards on to the floor.

Tips
This pose flexes the cervical spine significantly, placing stress on to the spinal tissues. To reduce flexion demands, perform the pose with your shoulders on a pad. This can be four yoga blocks or two or three folded yoga blankets of sufficient size for your shoulders to rest and not slip over the edge. Your head rests on the mat at a lower position than your shoulders, reducing the cervical flexion motion range.

Exercise 189 Inverted staff pose (Viparita Dandasana)

Tips

This is an intense stretch for the spine, chest and shoulders. It is important to move into and out of the pose in a controlled fashion and to progress the exercise gradually as your range of motion allows.

Purpose

To impart passive extension force on to the spine.

Preparation

Place a stack of yoga blocks against a wall, and sit on a chair or gym bench placed leg length away from the wall.

Action

- Lie supine on the chair seat with your feet flat on the floor. Shift your upper body up and down until the chair edge is in line with the lower part of your shoulder blade (inferior angle of scapula). Hold the chair frame for support and arch your spine backwards into extension over the chair seat edge. Lift your feet one at a time on to the blocks and straighten your legs, tightening your quadriceps muscles and pressing your heels downwards on to the blocks.
- Allow your head to lower downwards so the crown faces the floor. Reach your arms back and out to hold the lower frame of the chair.
- To increase motion range, place your heels on the floor rather than on blocks.

Exercise **190** Bridge (Setu Bandha)

- Perform action one and then bend your elbows placing your hands into your back on either side of the spine. Press with your hands to lift your chest. Once in the maximally lifted position straighten first one leg and then the other pressing your heels firmly into the ground and tightening your quadriceps muscles.
- To reduce the work on the arms, lift into the bridge position and place several foam blocks or a single wooden block (standing on end) beneath your pelvis. Straighten your legs, tightening your quadriceps and pressing your heels firmly into the floor, keeping your arms on the floor at the side of your body, palms facing up.

Tips

Placing your hands or support further up the spine focuses the extension movement into the thoracic spine in addition to the lumbar spine. The action is an intense extension stretch and it will take time for the spine to release into this position. Build the height of the support gradually over several exercise periods. The pose should be challenging but not painful.

Purpose

To strengthen and mobilise the spine into extension.

Preparation

Begin lying on your back with your knees bent and feet flat, arms by your sides, palms downwards.

Action

- Press down with your hands and feet and lift your hips so that you form a straight line from your shoulders through your hips, thighs and knees. Hold the position for three breaths and then slowly lower under control.

Exercise 191 Half-moon pose (Ardha Chandrasana)

Purpose

To stabilise the hips and spine while increasing flexibility of the leg and chest.

Preparation

Begin in the triangle pose (*see* page 263) with your left leg forward and left arm downwards gripping your left shin.

Action

*   To perform the classic half-moon pose (Ardha Chandrasana), begin in the triangle pose, reach your left hand away from your body (shoulder abduction) and place your hand on to the floor in line with your feet. Maintain your spinal alignment by adjusting your hand height. Take your hand higher by using your fingertips or placing your hand on to a yoga brick, and lower by placing the flat of your hands on to the floor. Raise your right leg, keeping it locked our straight, to the horizontal or in line with your spine. Ensure that your hips are 'stacked', that is the top hip is aligned directly over the bottom hip so that your pelvis faces forwards.
*   For the revolved half-moon pose (Parivrtta Ardha Chandrasana) begin by performing the revolved triangle (*see* page 263). Reach your leading (left) hand forwards to place it on to the floor directly beneath your shoulder (for beginners the hand can be placed in line with the inside edge of the foot rather than the outside edge). Press firmly against the floor and lift your straight left leg upwards to the horizontal. Turn your chest to the right and raise your right hand into the air.

Tips

The half-moon pose places intense demands on the hip stability of the weight-bearing leg. The bodyweight, multiplied by leverage due to the horizontal body position, must be taken on one hip. It is essential that you stabilise the hip by sucking the hip muscles in tightly (gluteus medius activity) and at the same time tightening the leg muscles (co-contraction of the quadriceps and hamstrings) to lock the knee. In those who have a tendency to hyperextend the knee (genu recurvatum) it is important that the hip, knee and ankle joints remain in vertical alignment (stacked) and the knee does not fall behind the limb line.

Exercise 192 Adepts or perfect pose (Siddhasana)

Purpose

To lengthen the tissues around the hip in an abducted and laterally rotated direction.

Preparation

Begin sitting on one or two yoga blocks to enable you to sit tall and maintain spinal alignment (normal lumbar lordosis).

Action

- Bend your left knee and draw your left foot in towards your groin, placing the top of your foot (dorsum) flat on to the mat. Bend your right knee and draw inwards in the same way, aiming to place one heel on top of the other, with the ankle bones (malleoli) one in front of the other. Allow your knees to relax downwards to rest on the floor.

Tips

You may place a folded towel or pad between your ankles to prevent bone pressing against bone.

Where your knees are very far off the ground, place yoga pads or cushions between them and the floor to take the weight of your legs and enable them to relax.

The exercise combines hip abduction, external rotation and flexion to release and lengthen the hip adductor and extensor muscles (buttock region) and hip joint tissues themselves. Although this is a useful action given that most sitting postures restrict full hip motion, there are two important considerations. First, seated poses in yoga are based on squatting actions which were traditionally used in many Indian cultures, but are less familiar to the Western lifestyle. Second, movement range at the hip may be limited by body shape, with asymmetry (one side different than the other) and changes in hip joint contour due to medical conditions (hip dysplasia). It is important that hip joint motion is encouraged, but never forced as injury to the joint may occur in the presence of underlying clinical conditions.

Exercise 193 Cobbler pose (Baddha Konasana)

Purpose
To lengthen the tissues around the hip in an abducted and laterally rotated direction, giving intense stretch.

Preparation
Begin sitting on a folded blanket or yoga block to enable you to sit tall and maintain spinal alignment (normal lumbar lordosis).

Action
- Draw the soles of your feet together and lower your knees to the floor. Hold your feet and gently pull them in towards your body, at the same time lengthening your spine to reach your head upwards towards the ceiling.
- Perform the above action, and press down with your elbows on to your thighs to encourage your legs to go lower.
- Use a contract-relax technique by pressing your thighs upwards against the downward pressure of your elbows (isometric hip adduction) and then release, pressing your legs down as your adductor muscle tone reduces.
- Angle your body forwards (trunk flexing on hip) by reaching your hands forwards along the floor and drawing your chest downwards. Try to maintain spinal alignment for as long as possible to avoid excessive spinal flexion. Allow your spine to flex only towards the edge of the movement and rest your head on two or three blocks.

Tips
This action combines lengthening into hip abduction and lateral flexion seen in the Adept's pose on page 279, with more extreme hip flexion by drawing the trunk downwards on a fixed thigh (femur). Focusing on spinal flexion (aiming the head to the floor) rather than on trunk flexion (moving the chest to the floor and keeping the head in line with the spine) can place excessive flexion stress on to the spinal tissues.

RECOMMENDED READING AND REFERENCES

RECOMMENDED READING

Bean, A., *The Complete Guide to Strength Training* (2nd edition) (A & C Black, London, 2001)

Enoka, R. M., *Neuromechanical Basis of Kinesiology* (3rd edition) (Human Kinetics, Champaign, Illinois, 2002)

Jones, K., and Barker, K., *Human Movement Explained* (Butterworth Heinemann, Oxford, 1996)

Kendall, F. P., McCreary, E. K., and Provance, P. G., *Muscles: Testing and Function* (Williams and Wilkins, Baltimore, 1993)

Levangie, P. K., and Norkin, C. C., *Joint Structure and Function* (3rd edition) (F. A. Davies, Philadelphia, 2001)

Norris, Christopher M., *Abdominal Training* (A & C Black, London, 1997)

Norris, Christopher M., *Back Stability* (Human Kinetics, Champaign, Illinois, 1999)

Norris, Christopher M., *Bodytoning*, (A & C Black, London, 2003)

Norris, Christopher M., *Sports Injuries, Diagnosis and Management* (3rd edition) (Butterworth Heinemann, Oxford, 2004)

Palastanga, N., Field, D., Soames, R., & Bogduk, N., *Anatomy and Human Movement: Structure and function* (Butterworth Heinemann, Oxford, 1994)

REFERENCES

Adams, M. A., Hutton, W. C., and Stott, J. R. R., 1980, 'The resistance to flexion of the lumbar intervertebral joint', Spine, 5: 245–253

Astrand, P. O., and Rodahl, K., 1986, *Textbook of Work Physiology*, McGraw-Hill, Maidenhead

Aveda, J., Kyrolainen, H., and Komi, P. V., 1999, 'Altered reflex sensitivity after repeated and prolonged passive muscle stretching', Journal of Applied Physiology, 86: 1283-1291

Bandy, W. D., and Irion, J. M., 1994, 'The effect of time on static stretch of the flexibility of the hamstring muscles', Physical Therapy, 74(9): 845–852

Barnard, H., Gardner, G. W., Diaco, N. V., MacAlpin, R. N., and Kattus, A. A., 1973, 'Cardiovascular responses to sudden strenuous exercise. Heart rate, blood pressure, and ECG', Journal of Applied Physiology, 34: 883–892

Bergh, U., 1980, 'Human power at subnormal body temperatures', ActaPhysiologica Scandinavia, 478 (supplement): 1–39

Bergh, U., and Ekblom, B., 1979, 'Physical performance and peak aerobic power at different body temperatures', Journal of Applied Physiology, 46: 885–889

Butler, D. S., 1991, *Mobilisation of the Nervous System*, Churchill Livingstone, Edinburgh

Carlson, C. R., Collins, F., Nitz, A., et al., 1990, 'Muscle stretching as an alternative relaxation training procedure', Journal of Behavior Therapy and Experimental Psychiatry, 21(1): 29–38

Castellote-Caballero, Y., Valenza, M., Martin-Martin, L., et al., 2013, 'Effects of a neurodynamic sliding technique on hamstring flexibility in healthy male soccer players: A pilot study', Physical Therapy in Sports, 14: 156–162

Cleland, J. A., Child, J. D., Palmer, J. A., and Eberhart, S., 2006, 'Slump stretching in the management of non-radicular low back pain: A pilot clinical trial', Manual Therapy, 11(4): 279–286

Dargent-Molina, P., Favier, F., Grandjean, H., et al., 1996, 'Fall-related factors and risk of hip fractures: the EPIDOS prospective study', The Lancet, 348: 145–149

Ekstrand, J., Gillquist, J., and Lilzedahl, S. S., 1983, 'Prevention of soccer injuries. Supervision by doctor and physiotherapist', *American Journal of Sports Medicine*, 11: 116–120

Engel, L., and Andersen L. B., 2000, 'Effects of body–mind training and relaxation stretching on persons with chronic toxic encephalopathy', *Patient Education and Counseling*, 39(2): 155–161

Enoka, R. M., 1994, 'Neuromechanical basis of kinesiology', *Human Kinetics*, Champaign, Illinois, USA

Etnyre, B. R., and Abraham, L. D., 1986, 'Gains in range of ankle dorsiflexion using three popular stretching techniques', *American Journal of Physical Medicine*, 65: 189–196

Fradkin, A. J., Gabbe, B. J., and Cameron, P. A., 2006, 'Does warming up prevent injury in sport? The evidence from randomised controlled trials', *Journal of Science and Medicine in Sport*, 9(3): 214–220

Gleim, G. W., Stachenfeld, N. S., and Nicholas, J. A., 1990, 'The influence of flexibility on the economy of walking and jogging', *Journal of Orthopaedic Research*, 8: 814–823

Godges, J. J., MacRae, H., and Longdon, C., 1989, 'The effects of two stretching procedures on hip range of motion and gait economy', *Journal of Orthopedic and Sports Physical Therapy*, 10(9): 350–357

Halbertsma, J. A., van Bolhuis, A. L., and Gloehen, L. N., 1996, *Archives of Physical Medicine and Rehabilitation*, 77: 688–692

IYUK (2013) Iyengar yoga teaching syllabus (Introductory levels 1 & 2), Iyengar yoga (UK), Crowborough, East Sussex, England

Jarvinen, T. A., Jozsa, L., Kannus, P., et al., 2002, 'Organisation and distribution of intramuscular connective tissue in normal and immobilized skeletal muscles', *Journal of Muscle Research and Cell Motility*, 23: 245–254

Johns, R. J., and Wright, V., 1992, 'Relative importance of various tissues in joint stiffness', *Journal of Applied Physiology*, 17: 824–828

Kabat-Zinn, J., 2007, *Full Catastrophe Living*, 15th edition, Piatkus, UK

LaBan, M. M., 1962, 'Collagen tissue: implications of its response to stress in vitro', *Archives of Physical Medicine and Rehabilitation*, 43: 461–466

Leelarungrayub, D., Pothongsunun, P., Yankai A., and Pratanaphon, S., 2009, 'Acute clinical benefits of chest wall-stretching exercise on expired tidal volume, dyspnea and chest expansion in a patient with chronic obstructive pulmonary disease: A single case study', *Journal of Bodywork and Movement Therapies*, 13(4): 338–343

Li, Y., McClure, P. W., and Pratt, N., 1996, 'The effect of hamstring muscle stretching on standing posture and on lumbar and hip motions during forward bending', *Physical Therapy*, 76: 836–845

Magnusson, S. P., Simonsen, E. B., and Kjaer, M., 1996, 'Biomechanical responses to repeated stretches in human hamstring muscle in vitro', *American Journal of Sports Medicine*, 24(5): 622–628

Marshall, P. W., Cashman, A., and Cheema, B., 2011, 'A randomized controlled trial for the effect of passive stretching on measures of hamstring extensibility, passive stiffness, strength, and stretch tolerance', *Journal of Science and Medicine in Sport*, 14(6) 535–540.

McNair, P. J., and Stanley, S. N., 1996, 'Effect of passive stretching and jogging on the series elastic muscle stiffness and range of motion of the ankle joint', *British Journal of Sports Medicine*, 30: 313–318

Millar, A. P., 1976, 'An early stretching routine of calf muscle strains', *Medicine and Science in Sports and Exercise*, 22(3): 632–641

Moore, M. A., and Kukulka, C. G., 1991, 'Depression of Hoffman reflexes following voluntary contraction and implications for proprioceptive neuromuscular facilitation therapy', *Physical Therapy*, 71: 321–333

Nelson, A. G., Kokkonen, J., and Arnall, D. A., 2005, 'Acute muscle stretching inhibits muscle strength endurance performance', *Journal of Strength and Conditioning Research*, 19(2): 338–343

Nicol, C., Komi, P. V., and Horita, T., 1996, 'Reduced stretch–reflex sensitivity after exhausting stretch–shortening cycle exercise', *European Journal of Applied Physiology*, 72: 401–409

Norris, C. M., 2011, *Managing Sports Injuries*, 4th Edition, Churchill Livingstone, Oxford

Norris, C. M., 1998, *Sports Injuries. Diagnosis and Management*, Butterworth Heinemann, London

Putt, M. T., Watson, M., Seale, H., and Paratz, J., 2008, 'Muscle Stretching Technique Increases Vital Capacity and Range of Motion in Patients With Chronic Obstructive Pulmonary Disease', *Archives of Physical Medicine and Rehabilitation*, 89(6):1103–1107

Rodackia, A. L., Souzaa, R., Ugrinowitschb, C., Cristopoliskia F., and Fowler, N., 2009, 'Transient effects of stretching exercises on gait parameters of elderly women', *Manual Therapy*, 14(2): 167–172

Rosenbaum, D., and Henning, E. M., 1995, 'The influence of stretching and warm-up exercises on Achilles tendon reflex activity', *Journal of Sports Science*, 15: 481–484

Safran, M. R., Garrett, W. E., Seaber, A. V., Glisson, R. R., and Ribbecsk, B. M., 1988, 'The role of warm-up in muscular injury prevention', *American Journal of Sports Medicine*, 16(2)

Samukawa, M., Hattori, M., Sugama, N., and Takeda, N., 2011, 'The effects of dynamic stretching on plantar flexor muscle-tendon tissue properties', *Manual Therapy* 16(6): 618–622

Schleip, R., Chaitow, L., Findley, T. W., and Huijing, P., 2012, *Fascia – The tensional network of the human body*, Elsevier, Edinburgh

Schleip, R., Jager, H., and Klingler, W., 2012, 'What is fascia? A review of different nomenclatures', *Journal of Bodywork and Movement Therapies*, 16: 496–502

Schleip, R., and Muller, D. G., 2013, 'Training principles for fascial connective tissues: Scientific foundation and suggested practical applications', *Journal of Bodywork and Movement Therapies*, 17: 103–115

Shrier, I., 2004, 'Does stretching improve performance? A systematic and critical review of the literature', *Clinical Journal of Sports Medicine*, 14(5): 267–273

Sullivan, M. K., Dejulia, J. J., and Worrell, T. W., 1992, 'Effect of pelvic position and stretching method on hamstring muscle flexibility', *Medicine and Science in Sports and Exercise*, 24: 1383–1389

Taylor, D. C., Dalton, J., Seaber, A. V, and Garrett, W. E., 1990, 'The viscoelastic properties of muscle-tendon units', *American Journal of Sports Medicine*, 18: 300–309

Thomas, J. R., and Nelson, J. K., 1990, second edition, *Research Methods in Physical Activity*, Human Kinetics, Champaign, Illinois, USA

Trampasa, A., Kitsiosa, A., Sykarasa, E., et al., 2010 'Clinical massage and modified Proprioceptive Neuromuscular Facilitation stretching in males with latent myofascial trigger points', *Physical Therapy in Sport*, 11(3): 91–98

Warren, C. G., Lehmann, J. F., and Koblanski, J. N., 1971, 'Elongation of rat tail tendon: effect of load and temperature', *Archives of Physical Medicine and Rehabilitation*, 51: 465–474

Watt, J. R., Jackson, K., Franz, J. R., et al., 2011, 'Effect of a Supervised Hip Flexor Stretching Program on Gait in Elderly Individuals', *PM&R*, 3(4): 324–329

Webright, W. G., Randolph, B. J., and Perrin, D. H., 1997, 'Comparison of nonballistic active knee extension in neural slump position and static techniques on hamstring flexibility', *Journal of Orthopedic and Sports Physical Therapy*, 26: 7–13

Williams, M., and Penman, D., 2011, *Mindfullness*, Piatkus, London

Witvrouw, E., Mahieu, N., Danneels, L., and McNair, P., 2004, 'Stretching and injury prevention: an obscure relationship', *Sports Medicine*, 34(7): 443–439

Young, W., Elias, G., and Power, J., 2006, 'Effects of static stretching volume and intensity on plantar flexor explosive force production and range of motion', *Journal of Sports Medicine and Physical Fitness*, 46: 403–411.

Zakas, A., Doganis, G., Papakonstandinou, V., et al., 2006, 'Acute effects of static stretching duration on isokinetic peak torque production of soccer players', *Journal of Bodywork and Movement Therapies*, 19: 8–9

INDEX OF EXERCISES

INDEX